Praise for *Healthy Places, Healthy People, Second Edition:
A Handbook for Culturally Informed Community Nursing Practice*

"*Healthy Places, Healthy People, Second Edition,* is a textbook that engages students on a journey of discovery into the multiple issues that impact health in the communities where their patients live."

–*Kathy Perzynski, MS, RN*
Associate Professor
Lourdes College, Sylvania, Ohio

"If you are looking for a textbook with a fresh, contemporary approach toward working with communities that truly takes into account the multiple determinants of health, this book is for you. *Healthy Places, Healthy People, Second Edition,* successfully integrates the concepts of community/public health nursing with culture in a meaningful and practical way. As a community health nurse educator with an expertise in culturally informed care, I would use this text for learners at all levels."

–*Donna Z. Shambley-Ebron, PhD, RN, CTN-A*
Associate Professor, University of Cincinnati

"Dreher and Skemp's offering goes beyond the usual community/public health nursing textbook to become a practical and useful guide for making healthy communities a reality. Moving away from health behaviors, the authors focus on the social and environmental determinants of health. This book will be useful for those educators who want to emphasize the role social justice has in creating a healthy society."

"*Healthy Places, Healthy People, Second Edition,* is an essential compendium of best practices, evidence-based solutions, tools, and formulas for nursing professionals as they engage with stakeholders—from insurance companies to primary care providers to hospital and academic medical centers—to navigate the climate of health care reform on behalf of individuals living in their community."

HEALTHY PLACES HEALTHY PEOPLE

SECOND EDITION

A Handbook for Culturally Informed Community Nursing Practice

Melanie Creagan Dreher, PhD, RN, FAAN
Lisa Elaine Skemp, PhD, RN

Sigma Theta Tau International
Honor Society of Nursing®

Sigma Theta Tau International

Copyright © 2011 by Sigma Theta Tau International

> The Honor Society of Nursing, Sigma Theta Tau International (STTI), is a nonprofit organization whose mission is to support the learning, knowledge, and professional development of nurses committed to making a difference in health worldwide. Founded in 1922, STTI has 130,000 members in 86 countries. Members include practicing nurses, instructors, researchers, policymakers, entrepreneurs, and others. STTI's 470 chapters are located at 586 institutions of higher education throughout Australia, Botswana, Brazil, Canada, Colombia, Ghana, Hong Kong, Japan, Kenya, Malawi, Mexico, The Netherlands, Pakistan, Singapore, South Africa, South Korea, Swaziland, Sweden, Taiwan, Tanzania, the United States, and Wales. More information about STTI can be found online at www.nursingsociety.org.

Sigma Theta Tau International
550 West North Street
Indianapolis, IN 46202

To order additional books, buy in bulk, or order for corporate use, contact Nursing Knowledge International TOLL FREE at 888.654.4968 (US and Canada) or +1.317.634.8171 (outside US and Canada).

To request a review copy for course adoption, e-mail solutions@nursingknowledge.org or call TOLL FREE at 888.654.4968 (US and Canada) or +1.317.634.8171 (outside US and Canada).

To request author information, or for speaker or other media requests, contact Rachael McLaughlin of the Honor Society of Nursing, Sigma Theta Tau International at 888.634.7575 (US and Canada) or +1.317.634.8171 (outside US and Canada).

ISBN: 978-1-935476-62-7
EPUB/Mobi ISBN: 978-1-935476-63-4
PDF ISBN: 978-1-935476-64-1

Library of Congress Cataloging-in-Publication Data

Dreher, Melanie Creagan.
  Healthy places, healthy people : a handbook for culturally informed community nursing practice / Melanie Dreher and Lisa Skemp. -- 2nd ed.
    p. ; cm.
  Includes bibliographical references.
  ISBN 978-1-935476-62-7 (alk. paper)
1. Community health nursing. 2. Community health services. I. Skemp, Lisa, 1955- II. Sigma Theta Tau International. III. Title.
  [DNLM: 1. Community Health Nursing. 2. Community Health Services. 3. Cultural Competency. 4. Transcultural Nursing--methods. WY 106]
  RT98.D74 2011
  610.73'43--dc23
                          2011019790

First Printing, 2011

Publisher: Renee Wilmeth
Acquisitions Editor: Janet Boivin, RN
Editorial Coordinator: Paula Jeffers
Interior Design and Page Composition: Rebecca Batchelor

Principal Editor: Carla Hall
Development Editor: Kate Shoup
Indexer: Johanna VanHoose Dinse
Cover Design: Rebecca Batchelor

Dedication

This book is dedicated to Professor Lambros Comitas, Teachers College, Columbia University, who taught us how communities work and how to work with communities.

ACKNOWLEDGEMENTS

We are deeply indebted to the communities in which we work and the people and groups that open their doors and hearts to our students and faculty. The University of Massachusetts, University of Iowa, and Rush University students, who embraced a new way to nurse and enthusiastically set about working with community members in creating healthier places for people to have healthier lives, also deserve our gratitude.

The genesis is easily traced to Columbia University Department of Anthropology and Professor Conrad Arensberg, whose concepts of community and culture are the foundation of our treatise, and we are deeply grateful for his wisdom. There are not sufficient ways to thank Kathy Pryzynski, Maureen Groden, Ken Culp, and Dayton Jacques for their thoughtful comments on this revised edition. We are especially grateful for the contributions of Dolores Shapiro and Michelene Asselin, the original co-authors of *Healthy Places, Healthy People*. And finally, we thank our families, friends, and colleagues for unrelenting patience and support.

–Melanie Creagan Dreher, PhD, RN, FAAN

–Lisa Elaine Skemp PhD, RN

About the Authors

Melanie Creagan Dreher, PhD, RN, FAAN

Melanie Dreher is the John and Helen Kellogg dean and professor at Rush University College of Nursing. An educator for more almost 40 years, Dreher has championed nursing as the profession with the greatest potential to improve the health and well-being of people in communities. She has taught community assessment, analysis, and intervention at Columbia University, University of Miami, University of Massachusetts, University of Iowa, and Rush University. After graduating from Long Island College Hospital, she earned her bachelor's degree in nursing at Long Island University and her doctorate in anthropology at Columbia University and Teachers College. Dreher's extensive ethnographic research in the Caribbean has focused on communities as powerful determinants of the health and welfare of children and adults. As a member of the charter Council of Public Representatives, she brought the realities of people living in communities to the National Institutes of Health. Currently, she brings her knowledge of communities and health to the Chicago Board of Health, the Trinity Health System Board of Directors, and the Board of Directors of Wellmark, Inc., Blue Cross Blue Shield of Iowa and South Dakota. Finally, she received a citation from the U. S. Ambassador for her community development work in Jamaica where she held a visiting professorship at the University of West Indies. Dreher has published extensively on culture as an organizing concept in nursing education and practice.

Lisa Elaine Skemp, PhD, RN

Lisa Skemp is currently Associate Professor of Adult and Gerontological Nursing at the University of Iowa College of Nursing and the Director of the Global Health Initiative at the Iowa Hartford Center of Geriatric Nursing Excellence. She will take over the Endowed Chair in Gerontological Nursing at Our Lady of the Lake College, a private college of the Franciscan Missionaries of Our Lady Health System located in Louisiana. In 2000 she received the American Public Health Association New Investigator's Award for her cross-cultural research in the Caribbean, and in 2003 she became a Claire M. Fagin Fellow for her work in rural, community based healthy aging. After receiving her BSN from Viterbo University, she obtained her master's degree in Community Health Nursing and Education and then her doctorate in nursing at the University of Iowa with an emphasis in community based gerontology. Skemp integrates her role as an educator in community health nursing and global health with her research and practice in diverse cultures and communities. Her extensive ethnographic research includes community based studies in St. Lucia, West Indies, rural American Midwest farming communities, Mexican immigrant populations, Sudanese refugee groups in Iowa, and South India tribal haddies. Professor Skemp's contributions to global health include development of the Gerontology Healthy Ageing Portal (GHAP) on the WiderNet eGranary Digital Library and two study abroad programs in interprofessional community capacity building for healthy aging in St. Lucia and South India. In affiliation with WHO, she convenes the Alliance for Healthy Active Aging (AHAA), an interprofessional virtual network.

TABLE OF CONTENTS

Introduction xv

1 The Cultural Framework of Community Health 1

    Why Culture? 2

        What Is Cultural Competence? 3

        Cultural Competence in Public Health 5

    What Is a Community? 7

        Physical Environment 7

        Population 8

        Social Organization 9

        Community: A Definition 10

    What Is Community Health? .10

    The Scientific Foundation of Community Health Nursing 12

        Epidemiology 12

        Anthropology 14

    Political Conservatism in Community Nursing 16

2 Culturally Informed Community Health Practice 19

    What Is Community/Public Health Nursing? 20

    The Community Health Legacy 20

    The Community Practice Paradigm 22

        Community Clients 22

        Community Practice Goals 24

        Community Assessment 26

        Community Planning and Intervention 27

        Community Coordination 30

        Community Evaluation 31

The Nurse-Community Relationship. 31

Community Nursing Values 33

3   Strategies for Entering and Understanding
    Your Community 35

    Knowing Your Community—Its Strengths, Its Issues,
    and Its Problems. 36

    Informing Public Health Practice through Epidemiology
    and Bio-Statistics 37

    Bio-Statistical Measures of Population Health *37*
    Calculating Rates *38*

    Epidemiological Studies of Population Health 43

    Case-Control Studies. *43*
    Cohort Studies *45*

    Informing Public Health Practice Through Anthropology
    and Ethnography. 48

    Understanding the Matrix of Health and Illness Through . . . .
    Ethnography *49*

    Gathering Community Data. 50

    What We Observe Directly About the Community *52*
    What People Tell Us About the Community *55*
    What Is Documented About the Community. *57*

    Accessing Public Health Data 60

    The United States Census. *60*
    The Centers for Disease Control and Prevention (CDC) *61*
    State Health Departments. *61*
    Local Sources. *62*
    Health Surveys and Epidemiological Studies *62*
    Internet Sources for Health Statistics *63*

Pulling It Together: Culturally Informed Community Health
Analysis 68

4   Discovering the Culture of Your Community 75

Community Culture Inquiry 76

The Physical Environment of a Community. 77
   Spatial Dimensions of Community Life. *77*
   Temporal Dimensions of Community Life *87*

The Population of a Community .93

The Social Organization of a Community 103
   Community Institutions. *103*
   Government, Politics, and Law Enforcement. *107*
   Horizontal Stratification. *118*
   Vertical Segmentation *120*

5   Determining the Health of Your Community 125

Community Health Assessment. 126

Environmental Health 126
   Toxic Substances and Hazardous Waste Management *132*
   Environmental Health Highlights. *149*

Population Health Assessment .150

Health Care Organization Assessment 166
   Prevention and Health Promotion *166*
   The Public Health Workforce *171*
   Information Systems *172*
   Public Health Agencies *172*
   Public Health Financing. *175*
   Indigenous and Alternative Health Systems *178*

6   Laying the Foundation for a Healthy Community
    Agenda. 181

    The Future is Now 182

    Why Is Planning So Important in Community
    Health Practice?. 183

    Health Planning: As It Was, Is, and Can Be 184
        Resource-Based Planning. 184
        Population-Based Planning 186
        Culture Based Planning 188

    Creating a Culturally Informed Healthy Community
    Agenda. 193
        Overarching Goals. 194
        Vision, Mission, and Values. 194
        Stakeholders and Community Engagement 196
        Objectives 198
        Strategies. 202

    Building a Constituency for Culture Based Action:
    Do We Need It? Who Should Be On It?. 205

7   Leading Culturally Informed Community Action 209

    Building Capacity Through Citizen Engagement. 210

    Guiding Change: A Culturally Preservative Approach 210

    Models for Action. 212

    The Role of the Nurse in Community Action. 216

    Creating an Action Plan for a Healthy Community Agenda. .218

The MAP-IT Framework: Mobilize, Assess, Plan,
Implement, Track 224

Mobilize *224*

Assess *226*

Plan *228*

Implement *230*

Track *231*

Formulating a Culturally Effective Community
Case Statement 237

References 241

Index 253

INTRODUCTION

This is the second edition of a book designed to help students of public health use the concept of culture to learn *how communities work* and *how to work with communities*. Like the first edition, this is not your standard textbook. Our goal is not a comprehensive survey of public health nursing. Our objective is to assist students in acquiring the *core public health leadership competencies* of community relationship building, inquiry, assessment, analysis, planning, action, evaluation, and persuasion that transcend the categorical public health concerns such as infectious diseases, maternal-child health, environment monitoring, and disaster preparedness. It is a small book with realistic strategies and practical advice on how to be more effective in mobilizing citizen action for public health. It contains useful tools for gathering, organizing, and analyzing community information to facilitate working with citizens and groups to build capacity for a healthy future. In many ways, it is a "how-to" book—a public health improvement strategy that can be applied to any community, at any time, to get the job of public health . accomplished.

The organizing theme of this edition has remained the same: **Healthy *places* are the building blocks for healthy *people*;** that is, the capacity of communities to assure a robust physical and social environment will promote and protect the health of their citizens. In this paradigm we make the distinction between *creating* health and *treating* health problems—a notion that often is not easily grasped by students who come to their course in public health fresh from the clinical imperatives of the acute care setting. Although access to quality clinical services and illness care is critically important (and disparities in access are symptomatic of an unhealthy community) we do not equate *health* with *health care*. It is in the cultural context of the community, stretching well beyond its clinics and hospitals, where the impact of social and environmental determinants is most keenly felt. Obvious examples include clean air, water, and land; safe highways; and uncontaminated food. But they also include the socioeconomic dislocations that place some members of a community on unequal footing—creating local "hot spots," that, left unattended, compromise the health of the whole community.

In this edition, we are perhaps even more strident about the powerful influence of *place* on health. Beginning, perhaps, with the Alameda County study in which human relationships took precedence over health behaviors as the number one predictor of mortality, new research continues to reveal the impact of residential *community culture* on health. In addition to the work of Roberts et al. cited in the first edition (and re-visited here), Bender, Clune, & Guruge, 2009; Carolan, Andrews, & Hodnett, 2006; Cummins, Stafford, Macintyre, Marmot, & Ellaway, 2005; Cummins, Curtis, Diez-Roux, & Macintyre 2007; Drevdahl 2002; Kerker, Bainbridge, Kennedy, Bennani, Agerton, et al., 2011; Kneipp & Drevdahl 2003; Marmot, 2005; 2009; Stafford & Marmot, 2003; Szwarcwald, da Mota, Damacena, & Pereira, 2011; and Tarlier, Browne, & Johnson, 2007, offer compelling evidence and justification for extending the examination of social and environmental determinants of health beyond the correlation of variables and into the situational realities of community context.

We also are loyal to the assertion put forward in the first edition that public health nursing is defined by *orientation* rather than by *setting*. The nurse who is employed in the cardiology clinic of a tertiary care setting and who sits on local and national policy boards for cardiac prevention, who speaks to women's groups throughout the community to educate them about the risks for heart disease in women, who establishes self-help programs for women with heart disease and links the families of women with cardiac pathology seen in the hospital to community services, has a strong *community health orientation*. In contrast, the nurse who is employed in a neighborhood-based prenatal clinic, but whose practice is limited to assessing and counseling expectant mothers, ignoring the obvious disparities in birth weight, the burden of parenthood, quality daycare programs, food and nutrition, transportation to the clinic, and existing regulations and housing policies that compromise the mothers' capacity to raise their children in a healthy and safe environment, might be working in a community setting but does not have a community orientation.

We contend the commonly made distinction between acute care and community care is spurious and diverts our attention from our true mission. The public does distinguish between care received in one system from that in another. The presence of a sufficient and well-integrated acute care system falls within the "assurance" responsibility of public health. Hospitals are simply another community institution, not unlike churches, schools, and factories, with an important role to play in promoting the health of the public. As public health providers, our goal is to offer a perspective that prepares *all* students for beginning practice in community health and to fulfill their responsibility for active citizenry. We do not distinguish between "community health nurse" and "public health nurse" and use the terms interchangeably throughout the book.

So what is different about this edition? First of all, the title. In both of the editions we have shared our concerns about the widespread misunderstanding of *culture* and the implications for *cultural competence*. Ultimately, we decided to end what seemed an inherent contradiction and have replaced the words "culturally competent" with "culturally informed." We also have avoided much reference to "vulnerable populations," one, because the term (like cultural competence) is so broadly used that it has lost its significance and, two, because it is a term that suggests dependency and weakness rather than the strength and opportunity that are waiting to be discovered and activated in a "culturally informed" community health practice.

Second, we took the advice of our readers who suggested we needed to do a better job of explaining ethnography as an anthropological method that could be used by nurses to understand both the health and culture of their communities. Our experience has been that concepts often are best comprehended by explaining what they are not, so beginning with Chapter 1, we juxtapose anthropology and epidemiology and their respective units of analysis—communities and populations—to illustrate the differences and the complementarities between the two scientific orientations in public health. Our readers also told us that our chapters on assessment in the first edition were long and somewhat tortuous, so we reorganized that material into three chapters that we believe better prepare students for their community entry and inquiry. To assist students to make the conceptual leap from the care of individuals to the care of whole communities, we also have included "suggested activities" throughout the book.

Third, in the first edition we referenced *Healthy People 2010* heavily. Now, *Healthy People 2020* has arrived. In addition to an excellent interactive website for students to learn how their communities compare with others nationally, it illustrates that public health is an interprofessional, community wide responsibility. But perhaps most importantly, *Healthy People 2020* is guided by two critical questions: (1) *What makes some people healthy and others unhealthy?* and (2) *How can we create a society in which everyone has a chance to live long healthy lives?* At a time when it is easy to be distracted by categorical problems, initiatives, and funding, we believe effective responses to these two great big societal questions requires a comprehensive and unrelenting focus on the health of the *whole* community and its culture.

Both *Healthy People 2010* and *2020* provide strategies for achieving their over arching goals. In 2010 three major categories of community interventions for promoting health were identified—educational, political, and environmental. *Healthy People 2020* added a project management model, called MAP-IT. With only three categories of interventions and a widely used logic model for planning and implementation, building capacity for community action would seem relatively straightforward. But inspiring communities to take action is not just formulating policies about the sale of cigarettes to minors or educating the public about the dangers of obesity or cleaning up a polluted river. When we start moving initiatives such as sex education or improving emission standards into the *cultural realities* of community life, things get much more complicated. Mobilizing specific *action* with a specific *population* in a specific *place* requires an understanding of the complexities of community culture, with all its diverse citizens, groups, interests, goals, and values that take us beyond *Healthy People 2020*.

The passage of the Patient Protection and Affordable Care Act in 2010, which extends access to 32,000,000 more Americans, provides unprecedented opportunities for nurses to fulfill their mandate to care for the health of the public (Institute of Medicine, 2010). Public health nurses will lead this change by assisting communities to discover their strengths and build the capacity necessary to shape the future of health and health care. Finally, in this edition, as in the first, we are committed to social justice and promoting the health of *all* people as enduring values. We embrace the promise of health reform not just for universal *access* to health services but for universal *engagement* in making communities welcoming environments in which to work, play, raise families, and experience long and healthy lives.

–Melanie Dreher, PhD, RN, FAAN

–Lisa Skemp, PhD, RN

THE CULTURAL FRAMEWORK OF COMMUNITY HEALTH

This chapter explains why culture is a critical organizing concept for community nursing practice. Drawing on methods from epidemiology and anthropology, it compares and contrasts the fundamental units of public health inquiry and practice—population and community—in relation to health and culture.

CHAPTER 1 OBJECTIVES

- Describe the significance of culture and community as organizing concepts in community nursing practice.

- Compare anthropology and epidemiology with regard to their units of analysis, strategies, and contributions for improving the public's health.

- Explain the ecological fallacy intrinsic to cultural competence, its application, and how it may impede care.

WHY CULTURE?

Culture is not a new concept in public health. The importance of knowing a community's culture to determine patterns of illness, health, and use of health services was documented almost 60 years ago in a landmark collection entitled *Health, Culture, and Community: Case Studies of Public Reactions to Health Programs* (Paul, 1955):

> If you wish to help a community improve its health, you must learn to think like the people. ... To assume new health habits, it is wise to ascertain the existing habits, how these habits are linked to one another, what functions they perform, and what they mean to those who practice them. (p. 1)

Nor is culture new for public health nurses. Over half a century ago, George Rosen (1954) advised:

> First and foremost comes a knowledge of the community and its people. This knowledge must be acquired and is just as important for successful public health work as is a knowledge of epidemiology or medicine. ... The community health nurse ... should be consciously aware of the way of life of the people, their goals in life, the motivations that make them do the things they do, the things in life that mean much or little to them. (p. 15)

Culture is a concept that distinguishes the practice of nursing from the practice of medicine (Dreher, 1996; Leininger, 1989). According to the American Nurses Association (2007):

> Nursing is the protection, promotion, and optimization of health and abilities, prevention of illness and injury, alleviation of suffering through the diagnosis and treatment of human response, and advocacy in the care of individuals, families, communities, and populations.

Unlike physicians, who treat a streptococcal infection in much the same manner in Bangkok as they would in London or use the same hip-replacement procedure in Kenya as in Canada, nurses must anticipate and accommodate the wide variation in a client's *response* to an infection or to post-surgical recovery. Nurses understand that individuals and families vary significantly in their responses not only to illness and injury, but to birth, death, disability, developmental transitions, treatment, and hospitalization, and that these variations are embedded in the context of home and community. To be most therapeutic, nurses must know more about their clients than just their disease, age, and sex. They must understand their clients' ways of life, values, education, occupation, social status, family responsibilities, and the meanings they have given to their illness.

Nursing, itself, is a cultural phenomenon, because most expressions of caring and comfort are responses learned in a cultural context and are subject to variation across ethnic and national groups. Similarly, to be effective in improving the health of the public, community nurses will want to know something more than the rate of HIV infection, the prevalence of diabetes, or the incidence of low–birth-weight babies. They also will want to know about the community's economy, religious institutions, educational resources, commonly held values, social norms, and justice systems, and the prevailing knowledge and beliefs about health, healing, and health care. In other words, nurses must understand the culture of the community to be served. Attention to culture exposes the range of personal, social, economic, and environmental factors that influence health status.

WHAT IS CULTURAL COMPETENCE?

Beginning with the groundbreaking work of Leininger (1989, 1997), culturally competent care has emerged as a mantra of contemporary nursing practice (Andrews and Boyle, 2008; Betancourt, Green, Carrillo, and Ananeh-Firempong, 2003; Campinha-Bacote and Munoz, 2001; Fahrenwald, Boysen, Fischer, and Mauer, 2001; USDHHS, 2001). Journals and books abound with formulas and instructions for students, educators, and clinicians on how to become more "culturally sensitive" and "culturally aware" in preparation for an increasingly diverse world. The underlying principle of cultural competence is that when patient care is guided by an understanding of cultural traditions, beliefs, and practices, patients and families will be more engaged, clinical outcomes will be improved, and efficiencies will occur.

As the world continues to evolve as a multi-ethnic, global society, an understanding and application of culture in all human services is wholesome, desirable, and consistent with principles of social justice. The quest for cultural competence, however, has not achieved its desired objectives in terms of widespread and routine incorporation of culture as a component of care for all patients (Benkert, Tanner, Guthrie, Oakley, and Pohl, 2005; Omeri and Malcolm, 2004; Williamson and Harrison, 2010). One reason for the disappointing results of the cultural competency movement is the opinion—widely shared among health professionals—that consideration of culture is necessary only when working with patients from other societies or "ethnic communities." Even more problematic, however, is a lack of understanding of the distinction between ethnicity as an individual characteristic and culture as a group characteristic. Ethnicity is a term used to connote traits associated with a common cultural, linguistic, behavioral, or religious ancestry. Jewish, Midwestern, Polish, and Hispanic are examples of ethnic identities. Culture, on the other hand, is a characteristic that refers to the learned patterns of behavior and beliefs passed on through generations of a specific group. It includes ways of life, norms and values, social institutions, customs, celebrations, and a shared construction of the physical world. Individuals go through life assuming only some features of the group to which they are born. Some might embrace the norms of their culture, while others might reject them; still others might apply them in some situations and not in others. Thus, it is common for individuals with the same ethnic background to exhibit varying levels of adherence to traditional cultural norms.

The distinction between culture as a group characteristic and ethnicity as an individual characteristic is important because in clinical practice, patient care is typically dispensed to individuals. When information about groups (cultures) is used to make decisions about individuals (clients), it is termed an *ecological fallacy* (Bernard, 2011; Clancy, Burger, and Magliozzi, 2003; Dreher and MacNaughton, 2002).

Ironically, in an attempt to be culturally competent, nurses and physicians often act on information that may not apply to specific individuals and could even compromise clinical effectiveness. If, for example, the normative definition of female physical beauty in a particular culture were five feet tall and 180 pounds, it would be easy to dismiss obesity in women as simply a cultural phenomenon and ignore the possibility of physiological or psychological pathology. Cultural norms regarding desired female body mass may, in fact, help explain the presence of obesity in a particular group, but they cannot be presumed to account for obesity in a particular woman. To treat this woman effectively, we still need to know whether, and to what extent, her obesity is attributable to cultural, physiological, or psychological factors, or their combination.

Finally, in addition to having a narrow conception of culture and making assumptions about cultural uniformity, we often fail to account for culture change. Although cultures differ in the speed at which change occurs and the degree of internal variation, few could be described as static and/or homogenous. Cultures are fluid and constantly respond to physical, social, economic, and political circumstances. As such, we must reject views of culture as monolithic and unchanging along with the widespread assumptions that people are "frozen" in cultural traditions, unable to modify their behavior and learn new ways.

CULTURAL COMPETENCE IN PUBLIC HEALTH

Although the concept of culture must be used judiciously in clinical practice, it is a potent and far-reaching concept in public health, when communities (groups) rather than individuals become the unit of intervention (Edelson, 2008; Fahren-wald et al., 2001; Kreuter and McClure, 2004; Racher and Annis, 2007). There-fore, while knowing the norms and beliefs regarding female beauty in a specific culture may not be useful for diagnosing the cause of obesity in individual patients, it may be of great value in designing effective responses to obesity in specific populations. It also would have theoretical value in explaining the social determinants of obesity. Knowledge of the social rules, norms, and patterns of behavior pertaining to food, nutrition, eating patterns, and preferred body size provide guidance for social marketing, public education programs, community based health promotion initiatives, and the organization of system level services. The most successful public health initiatives and community based programs are targeted to specific social groups, engage community leaders, and work with and through local institutions and established channels of communication (Tripp-Reimer, Choi, Skemp-Kelley, and Enslein, 2001). There is a commonly held opinion that partnerships for community action are greatly improved when health care providers and community residents are of the same ethnic and language group, minimizing cultural barriers to community action. Although it is easy to see why that assumption exists, there is ample evidence that cultural hurdles are attributable not so much to the lack of shared experience as they are to a failure to build meaningful relationships. If the health of a community is entrusted to individuals who have all the right education and credentials but who lack a relationship with those whom they are supposed to serve (Drevdahl, 1995), it will be difficult to formulate and achieve the goals of a healthy community agenda.

> In the H1N1 flu epidemic of 2010, when it was important first to immunize those most at risk (children and pregnant women), health departments did not have to go from house to house to ensure that immunizations were carried out effectively and efficiently. Instead, they deployed the communities' cultural capital (radio, newspapers, Internet, primary schools, faith institutions, after-school programs, neighborhood pharmacies, city colleges, hospital emergency rooms, teachers, volunteers, obstetricians, and primary-care providers) to ensure that women and children would be protected first.

Using a culturally informed approach (rather than a culturally competent approach), effective relationship-building is grounded in an understanding and appreciation of the community's cultural capital. *Cultural capital* is the arsenal of institutions, leaders, customs, knowledge, and values that forms the context for action and can be used to promote healthy, invested communities (Hopkins and Mehanna, 2000, 2003). The ultimate measure of whether public health intervention is culturally informed is the extent to which the community's cultural capital is deployed to protect and promote the health and well-being of its citizens.

WHAT IS A COMMUNITY?

Community is a broadly used term that can be applied to almost any configuration of people whose common values, characteristics, and/or interests unite them in some way (for example, a religious community, a retirement community, a community of undergraduate nursing students, or a community of scholars). Because community is a highly subjective concept, there are no correct or incorrect definitions, but some are more or less useful for a culturally informed public health practice. The broad applications of the term often do not capture the relationship between people and their habitat, which is the major concern of public health.

The concept of community is most useful for public health when it includes the following:

- The physical environment (spatial and temporal)

- The population (biological, social, and behavior characteristics of the people)

- The social organization or the ways in which the people of a community relate to each other through beliefs, values, and class structures, group affiliations, and institutions (Arensburg, 1954; Arensburg and Kimball, 1965)

It is not necessary for every citizen in a community to know every other citizen or to share cultural beliefs and values, but the members of a community must have a degree of intensity in their relationships with each other that distinguishes them from those outside of the community.

PHYSICAL ENVIRONMENT

The first dimension of communities is the manner in which they deploy the location in which the population resides and interacts and give it meaning (Arensburg, 1961; Drevdahl, 2002). The physical environment or context has two components:

■ **Spatial:** The spatial dimension includes the geophysical and climate factors, regional position, size, boundaries, land use, residential patterns, and manner in which people communicate and move (transport) from one area to another.

■ **Temporal:** In addition to communities occupying space, they also occupy time, using the hours of the day and days of the week, months, and years differently for different human functions—working, schooling, eating, celebrating, and so on.

Some communities are very much like they were 100 years ago, while others have changed dramatically. In the late 19th century, for example, communities grew and flourished at each stop of a burgeoning railway system. With the introduction of automobile transportation in the 1930s, however, families moved to new and larger homes on the outskirts. Schools, hospitals, and businesses followed, gradually replacing the small shops and services that had once served to bring the population together. Knowing the history of a community, its people, and its health is essential for predicting and planning for the future.

POPULATION

The population of a community is composed of the people who live or spend significant time there. The more general use of the term *population*, however, simply refers to any category of people who share one or more designated characteristic (for example, age, sex, eye color, residence, political orientation, occupation, disability, or religion). The population of a community, for example, consists of all those individuals who share the common characteristic of residence in or affiliation with a designated place (town, neighborhood, city, county, or country) at a particular point in time. The population of Cloudcroft, New Mexico, for example, is the aggregate number of people who reside within the established geopolitical boundaries of Cloudcroft. Within Cloudcroft, however, there may be a population of retired persons, a population of people with diabetes, and a population of Christians.

Unlike the more inclusive concept of community, a population is an objective reality and exactly equal to the sum of its parts based on the number of individuals included in the population. Therefore, if the number of people residing in Cloudcroft could be tabulated at a precise moment in time, it would be the same, no matter who measured it. In reality, of course, the size and characteristics of the population of Cloudcroft—or any village, city, state, or country—can change momentarily as residents are born, die, or migrate in or out. Within the last decade, for example, the ethnic composition of New Mexico has seen a 24.6% increase in Hispanic or Latino composition, recorded as 46.3% of the total population in 2009 (http://2010census. gov/2010census/data/).

> Although community is a more inclusive concept than population because it contains additional elements (social organization and environment), it is possible for populations to include many communities and for communities to include many populations.

SOCIAL ORGANIZATION

A community is not just a collection of people occupying the same space at the same time. Social organization turns a population and a place into a community. It implies that residents relate to one another in identifiable ways that distinguish them from those who are *not* of the community.

Social organization consists of institutions, belief systems, and cycles of activity that bring community members together for specific purposes such as religion, education, or commerce in discernable patterns and rhythms of work, play, and domestic activity according to the day, week, and season of the year. Residents, for example, may attend the same schools, work for the same employers, live in the same apartment building, or exercise at the same health club.

Although it is not necessary for all members of the community's population to hold the same beliefs, share the same values, or engage in the same behavior, social organization ensures that there are values and rules that generally guide the way people behave and interact with one another. These values and rules are passed through generations of families and individuals who enjoy varying levels of adherence to traditional norms and values.

COMMUNITY: A DEFINITION

For public health practice, we will define *community* as a place in which residents interact with each other and with their environment through a defined social organization. As culture carriers, communities are the lens through which we begin to understand the local context in which manifestations of health and illness are embedded. People do not live out their lives in populations. Nor do they live out their lives in cultures. Rather, people are born, grow, and experience health and illness in communities where circumstances generate conflict, where people do not always follow the rules, and where cultural norms and institutions fluctuate according to the exigencies of daily life. Communities take on a life of their own, with the capacity to change over time, independent of any one member. And because a community is bigger than the sum of its parts, it has a greater capacity for producing health than a single individual. Communities are where health and illness are produced and expressed, relationships are developed, plans are made, cultural capital is harnessed, and effective intervention occurs to build the community's capacity for health.

WHAT IS COMMUNITY HEALTH?

Understanding the community's environment, population, and social organization is necessary for understanding the community's health. A community's health is the result of a complex interaction between the population and its environment, mitigated by the social organization. In this ecological perspective, a public health problem reflects not just a problem with residents or a problem with their environment, but rather a problem in the relationship between the people and the place where they live, work, and play. To make it even more complex, human populations and environments change continuously; therefore, constant adaptation and re-adaptation are required to create and maintain healthy communities. Just as one health problem is resolved, new ones emerge to take its place. Milio (1975) put it succinctly: "Health is not a 'state' to be captured and dealt with;

nor is it some achievement to be attained with finality. It is rather the response of people to their environment" (p. 3).

Although this perspective suggests the quest for health as an outcome is futile, a "father" of contemporary public health, Rene Dubos (1965), advised that while health is a goal that is ever changing, it is nonetheless one toward which we must continue to strive through new discoveries and new solutions to health problems:

> In the world of reality, places change and man also changes. Furthermore, his self-imposed striving for ever-new distant goals makes his fate even more unpredictable than that of other living things. For this reason health and happiness cannot be absolute and permanent values, however careful the social and medical planning. Biological success in all its manifestations is a measure of fitness, and fitness requires never-ending efforts of adaptation to the total environment, which is ever changing. (p. 29)

Health as a continuously changing relationship between populations and their environment is easily grasped when common public health problems of the past, such as scurvy and smallpox, are compared with those of more-recent years, such as motor-vehicle accidents, drug abuse, school violence, nuclear disaster, terrorism, and HIV/AIDS (Gehlbach, 2005). In Healthy People 2020, 13 new foci were added to the list of achievable objectives, demonstrating increased public concern about the underrepresented populations of children and adolescents; older adults; and lesbian, gay, bisexual, and transgender people. Additional new topics include social determinants of health, global health, disaster preparedness, health related quality of life and well-being, blood disorders and blood safety, genetics, the dementias, sleep health, and health care associated infections.

To determine whether a community is healthy, we must look beyond the better-off citizens and neighborhoods and include an assessment of its poorest and most disenfranchised members. Nor can the health of a community be determined by averaging the measures of health across the community. The presence of any inequalities or disparities in the community puts the health of all community members at risk and offers the greatest challenges for public health. The term "disparities" refers to health conditions or outcomes that are associated with some kind of disadvantage. During the past decade, the elimination of health disparities was one of only two overarching goals for Healthy People 2010. Healthy People 2020 further expanded the health disparity goal to achieving health equity:

> ... the attainment of the highest level of health for all people. Achieving health equity requires valuing everyone equally with focused and ongoing societal efforts to address avoidable inequalities, historical and contemporary injustices, and the elimination of health and health care disparities. (USDHHS, Office of Minority Health, 2010).

This revised goal reflects the shift from the absence of disease as a measure of health to a focus on physical, mental, and social well-being. Just because there is not a disparity in disease, it does not automatically follow that there is no disparity in health.

THE SCIENTIFIC FOUNDATION OF COMMUNITY HEALTH NURSING

Traditionally, the fundamental science of public health has been epidemiology. Grounded in the notion that the individual is the basic unit of society, epidemiology identifies variations among populations in the distribution of health and environmental data to understand the probable etiology of diseases. On the other hand, medical anthropology focuses on the study of whole communities as the context for understanding the way in which culture influences health and illness. This section discusses the complementary nature of these two disciplines as the scientific foundation of community health nursing.

EPIDEMIOLOGY

In the last century, epidemiology has done more to enhance the health of the public through identification of risk factors and disease prevention than all the efforts of clinical medicine. Epidemiological research identifies variations among populations in the distribution of health problems to determine patterns and causes of disease. Using the individual, aggregated in populations, as the basic unit of inquiry, variables associated with a particular disease are identified as risk factors and are then associated with other risk factors. A simple and well-known example is the identification of tobacco-smoking as a risk factor for lung cancer. The goal of public health is to reduce the incidence and prevalence of lung cancer by reducing the incidence and prevalence of tobacco-smoking.

> At the time of this writing, our smallest state, Rhode Island, has the highest tax on cigarettes, at $3.46 per pack. If public health efforts were able to set and reach a public health goal of reducing the number of Rhode Island cigarette-smokers by 50,000, assuming the average smoker consumes one pack per day, the state would stand to lose $63,145,000 in annual revenues that support health care, education, and highway improvements.

With increasing recognition of the influence of cultural and social determinants on health and illness, epidemiological studies have expanded the usual biological risk factors (age, sex, and race) to include social and cultural determinants such as class, occupation, income, and education. Culture, as a group characteristic, has been approached as an individual risk factor—usually ethnicity or national origin. Being African American, for example, is considered a risk factor for hypertension; being American Indian is a risk factor for diabetes. Such correlations, however, do not distinguish ethnicity, an individual trait or characteristic, from culture, a group characteristic that describes community level patterns of beliefs, behaviors, and institutions. Taken out of context, these ethnic correlations do not explain how identified risk factors are connected in the complex neighborhoods, villages, and towns where people live out their daily lives. What are the factors, for example, that account for some American Indians being at greater risk for diabetes than other American Indians, or some African Americans being at greater risk for hypertension than other African Americans?

Public health would be easy if just knowing that tobacco-smoking and lung cancer are highly correlated were sufficient for people to discontinue cigarette-smoking and reduce the incidence and prevalence of lung cancer and other pulmonary diseases. To be effective community practitioners, we have to understand the cultural significance of smoking cigarettes and the political strength of the tobacco industry. We also have to know the economic impact of smoking cessation for people who earn a living growing tobacco and producing and distributing cigarettes as well as for the municipal and state governments that depend on cigarette taxation as a revenue stream. A successful anti-smoking campaign, for example, may reduce tobacco consumption among teenagers, but it may have little effect on ensuring the health of the community because local industry has not been persuaded to comply with recommended clean-air emission standards.

ANTHROPOLOGY

Unlike epidemiologists, medical anthropologists study whole communities to understand the constellation of local conditions on health and illness. Using ethnographic methods such as participant observation, kinship analysis, institutional analysis, and network analysis, anthropologists approach culture not as an individual risk factor (ethnicity) but as "the matrix of collective influences that shape the lives of groups and individuals" (Corin, 1994, p. 101). We have begun to have a better understanding of the importance of communities for growing and sustaining healthy people. The results of an early and well-known study of mortality in Alameda County, California (Berkman and Syme, 1979) revealed the most significant predictor of mortality was not among the predictable risk factors of smoking, diet, and exercise, but rather the extent to which individuals were socially connected within their families and communities.

With the development of medical anthropology as a discipline, there has been a mounting awareness that the relationship between health status and social status cannot be explained solely with reference to genetic variables, lifestyle choices, or differences in access to health services (Corin, 1994; Dressler, 1982, 1985, 2004). Rather, health inequalities are rooted in community culture, where the conditions of disparities are most evident and where determinants of health are embedded in the social and economic dislocations of residential communities (Cummins, Curtis, Diez-Roux, and Macintyre, 2007; Cummins, Stafford, Macintyre, Marmot, and Ellaway, 2005). When epidemiological studies and bio-statistical data regarding health disparities are reexamined in the light of ethnographic studies of single communities, the capacity of the community to engage its citizens in a network of health promoting social relationships also is revealed.

> A study of low infant birth weight in six Chicago neighborhoods demonstrated that neighborhood characteristics such as housing costs, crowding, community age distributions, and cultural homogeneity were more predictive of inequalities in maternal-infant health than individual risk factors such as race, ethnicity, and socioeconomic status. Surprisingly, neighborhoods with more middle-class housing had a *higher* rate of low infant birth weight than neighborhoods with more crowded housing and a higher concentration of young African-American residents (Roberts, 1997). These findings were explained by better social support for pregnant women in the more crowded but culturally homogenous neighborhoods and by the availability of more disposable income (for food and care) in neighborhoods with lower-cost housing.

Nurses, with their intimate and comprehensive knowledge of community life, are extraordinarily well positioned to collect and interpret cultural information about their communities. Although the mission of public health nurses is different from that of researchers, the description of the role of anthropologists in global health also describes the role of community health nurses (Helman, 2007):

- To ensure the cultural relevance of public health programs
- To identify community resources
- To monitor the impact of community interventions
- To mobilize expertise for health planning and implementation
- To influence policy-makers
- To advocate for communities at state, national, and international levels
- To continuously develop better, more-efficient ways to assess communities

POLITICAL CONSERVATISM IN COMMUNITY NURSING

We cannot leave this introductory chapter without reference to what could be called the ethos of community health nursing practice. Nursing's interest in culture emerged at the turn of the 20th century as public health nurses reported differences in life and health patterns between existing communities and immigrant communities. Later, when nursing education shifted from hospitals to universities, increased exposure to social sciences, such as anthropology, sociology, and political science, permitted nursing students to acquire a broader understanding of the determinants of health and illness. These include the social and economic dislocations that keep some communities on uneven footing, creating inequalities and disparities in health and health care.

Instead of using cultural knowledge to generate the "culturally transformative" (Tripp-Reimer *et al.*, 2001) far-reaching reform that could ameliorate some of the major health problems of society, nurses typically have limited their role in the promotion of health and prevention of disease to encouraging people to adopt healthy lifestyle behaviors. Notwithstanding the brilliant and courageous political activism of Lillian Wald, the founder of public health nursing, the profession, generally speaking, has not embraced the kind of system level action in the public arena required to address the myriad of daily assaults on healthy living experienced by some populations. These include inadequate housing, unsafe waste disposal, and dangerous traffic patterns. Even the most committed and passionate advocates for individual community residents are no match for the powerful forces that perpetuate inequality in health and access to care and allow the conditions of poor public health to exist.

Chafey (1996) addressed this problem in a critique of "caring" in its application to public health:

> Nurses must care about what happens to *groups* [sic] of citizens,
> as well as particular clients. ... Although proponents of "caring"
> seem to have drawn a distinction between an ethic of justice and
> an ethic of care, this is bipolar, even antithetical. Building the

health of communities requires universal application of the principles of justice. It further requires that nurses care enough about
their communities and the individuals in them to do battle in
political, social, and economic arenas. (p. 15)

The political conservatism that has characterized nursing has been attributed to
the socialization of nurses into passive roles and their lack of assertiveness. A
more probable explanation, however, lies in the nursing profession's almost exclusive concentration on individuals and families as the unit of nursing care. Typically, nursing education emphasizes nurse-patient and nurse-family relationships.
As a result, there are many excellent clinicians who are not necessarily well prepared to function in the public or political arena. With the exception of culture,
which often is misapplied in the care of individuals, nursing education generally
does not include theories that apply to group or community level behavior
(Dreher, 1982a, 2002; Drevdahl, 1995, 2002; Fahrenwald, Taylor, Kneipp, and
Canales, 2007; Tripp-Reimer, 1999). This is both a cause and a result of the traditional focus on individual care. Even in community nursing, theories grounded
in psychology (for example, anomie, symbolic interaction, cognitive dissonance,
and health belief models) continue to dominate nursing education and practice
along with the emphasis on personal health services.

Without an arsenal of theories and experiences that recognize whole communities
as a fundamental unit of public health service, nurses have been unequipped to
take group-level action. Formal definitions of community health nursing identifying geopolitically based populations as the unit of service are widely endorsed.
Yet, despite a continuing critique spanning thirty years (Butterfield, 1990, 2002;
Dreher, 1982a; Dreher and MacNaughton, 2002; Drevdahl, 1995; Fahrenwald *et
al.* 2007), students of community health nursing have limited opportunity to go
beyond assessment to community action—essential to distributive justice, equity,
and a just distribution of health resources (Levy and Sidel, 2006). Grounded in
principles of social justice and community self-determination, a brilliant and time-
less example of what nurses can do when they focus on creating healthy communities and not just on personal health services is presented in *9226 Kercheval
Street* (Milio, 1970):

While working as a young visiting nurse in an inner-city community in Detroit, Michigan, Milio discovered the most effective assistance she could provide to the mothers on public assistance was to help them be independent wage earners. To do this, she partnered with those mothers to establish a cooperative daycare center where they could safely leave their children while they entered the workforce. Fighting many political and financial battles, Milio helped her clients to initiate a daycare center and run it independently. Fundamentally, she engaged citizens in community level action in which they identified and deployed community cultural capital to create a healthier, more wholesome environment for children and their mothers.

Guided by the overarching goals of Healthy People 2020, this book is committed and designed to prepare students to work with whole communities and to take system level action to address the pressing and continuing disparities in health and health care (Fahrenwald, Taylor, Kneipp, and Canales, 2007). It is based on three premises:

- Health is a basic human right of all citizens.

- Healthy communities are the first and essential step to healthy people.

- Public health nurses are accountable for system level action to ensure social justice.

These premises are consistent with and guided by the overarching goals of Healthy People 2020:

- To attain high-quality, longer lives free of preventable disease, disability, injury, and premature death

- To achieve health equity, eliminate disparities, and improve the health of all groups

- To create social and physical environments that promote good health for all.

- To promote quality of life, healthy development, and healthy behaviors across all life stages.

2

CULTURALLY INFORMED COMMUNITY HEALTH PRACTICE

Although the notion of having a whole community as a client may be daunting at first, there is a culturally informed systematic approach for working with communities to achieve public health goals. It will require, however, a different way of thinking and a different set of skills. This chapter introduces community health nursing practice, exploring its distinctive features and explaining its guiding concepts, units of intervention, methods of assessment and action, nurse-client relationships, and guiding values.

CHAPTER 2 OBJECTIVES

- Within a historical context, identify the goals and unique features of community health nursing.

- Explain how community and population work together as guiding concepts in community health nursing.

- Specify the advantages of a community practice paradigm.

- Understand the significance of the nurse-community relationship.

- Describe the assumptions, ethics, and values of public health practice.

WHAT IS COMMUNITY/PUBLIC HEALTH NURSING?

Community health nursing differs from other kinds of practice in two important ways:

- The unit of practice is the whole community.

- The objective of practice is to promote and protect the health of the public.

These two features—communities as clients and the emphasis on health—are related in important ways. Caring for the health of the public requires community level intervention. By identifying and using a community's strengths, public health nurses work with residents and groups to promote and protect the health of the public.

THE COMMUNITY HEALTH LEGACY

The tradition for community/public health nursing was established in Liverpool, England, during the Victorian age, with the support of William Rathbone, a wealthy merchant and social reformer. On the advice of Florence Nightingale, Rathbone opened a training school in 1862 to prepare district nurses to oversee the health of designated communities. Meanwhile, American nursing activists, with the assistance of prominent women who had been to England and were strongly influenced by the work of Rathbone and Nightingale, began to institute district nursing in the United States. By the time Lillian Wald, the founder of public health nursing in the United States, established the Henry Street Settlement in New York City in the 1890s (Feld, 2008; Henry Street Settlement, n.d.), district-nursing organizations already had been established in several American cities.

These community health services, modeled after those in Great Britain, were available to the entire population in a designated area. A young Lillian Wald acknowledged the importance of prevention as she practiced nursing in the immigrant Jewish communities. She contended that all people, whether sick or ill, should receive health services (Buhler-Wilkerson, 1993). Starting as a volunteer, she and her colleagues educated residents of the Lower East Side in New York City about how diseases were transmitted and how to control infection. In her book *Windows on*

Henry Street (1934), Wald explains, "Our experience in one small East Side section, a block perhaps, had led to a next contact, and a next, in widening circles, until our community relationships have come to include the city, the state, the national government, and the world at large." (p. 167) In addition to establishing a visiting nurse service, Wald established a school nurse program to attend to the health needs of school age children and their families, and eventually introduced housing, education, employment assistance, and community recreational programs. Wald understood that the fundamental changes required to improve the health and welfare of poor immigrants could not be accomplished by a visiting program alone. She lobbied for health inspections of the workplace and for on-site health professionals to protect workers from unsafe conditions, she persuaded President Theodore Roosevelt to create a Federal Children's Bureau, and she convinced the New York Board of Education to hire its first nurse. In 1912, Wald helped found the National Organization for Public Health Nursing and served as its first president.

Following these early examples scattered throughout the major cities of the United States, district nursing also was brought to rural areas, mainly through the efforts of voluntary organizations such as the American Red Cross. Universal service to the entire community was the hallmark of district nursing. After the turn of the century, however, there was a marked shift toward specialization in public health nursing. This was prompted by a trend toward disease-oriented categorical funding programs, such as tuberculosis control and management of sexually transmitted infections. Formerly generalists, district nurses took on specialized roles in the care of individuals with particular health problems. With the exception of rural areas, universal service was gradually relinquished and replaced by an increasing concentration on *categorical* programs, such as programs to control communicable disease, and on special populations, such as pregnant women.

With the advent of Medicare funding, even rural communities were convinced to give up the comprehensive health promotion services of district nurses and replace them with illness care to specific individuals provided by home health nurses from a centralized visiting-nurse association (Dreher, 1984). Whether public community health nurses should be generalists, providing comprehensive services to the whole community, or specialists, providing illness care to individuals at home, has been debated for many decades. According to the Quad Council of Public Health Nursing Organizations (2004), there are two levels of community/public health competencies: the staff nurse generalist and the manager/specialist/consultant.

THE COMMUNITY PRACTICE PARADIGM

Caring for a whole community requires thinking about nursing in a different way. To better understand community health nursing, it is useful to compare the practice of nurses engaged in the care of whole communities to promote public health with that of nurse clinicians engaged in the care of individuals and families to prevent and manage illness.

COMMUNITY CLIENTS

Being responsible for the health of a whole town, county, or city neighborhood clearly distinguishes public health from clinical practice, but is the client a population or a community? In Chapter 1, "The Cultural Framework of Community Health," you learned that while the words "community" and "population" often are used interchangeably, communities and populations are not the same. Community is a more inclusive concept because it embraces not only populations, but the dynamic interplay of populations, environment, and social organizations. It is possible, however, for populations to include many communities and for communities to include many populations.

In reality, populations and communities are just different ways of looking at the same people. In public health, they are complementary perspectives for monitoring and protecting the health of the public, but it is critical to understand the difference and why both are important.

Suggested Activity

Using the definition of community in Chapter 1, identify populations within your community and name communities within your population.

Populations, the unit of analysis in epidemiology, are necessary for monitoring the health status of the people who reside and work in the community. Like offering K–12 education, maintaining roads, and providing protective services, public health is an official responsibility of government. To achieve accountability and comprehensiveness, public health services generally are organized according to geopolitically defined populations such as towns, cities, and counties, rather than by communities. Tracking the collective health of the people residing in these geopolitical units through bio-statistics and epidemiological surveys enables us to address the health needs of all citizens. Population health helps us to identify the magnitude of health problems, reveal correlations of disease and disability with population characteristics, designate those most at risk, and track the effectiveness of public health action.

One of the objectives of Healthy People 2020 is to increase the rate of immunization coverage among non-institutionalized adults 65 years of age and older to 90%. To do this effectively, both population data and community cultural data are required. It is important to know, at the very least, the size of the population over 65 years old, the number of cases of flu reported each year, and the number of those immunized to determine whether the 90% goal has been achieved. To make the program effective, however, it is important to know the role and status of elders in the specified communities and where they fit in community life (that is, where they live, where and when they get together, how often and for what purposes). With this information, community health teams can be more useful and efficient by incorporating the times and places in which elders in the community already routinely come together—for example, senior centers, local restaurants, libraries, religious centers, bingo games, and golf clubs. Such cultural knowledge reduces the costs of launching programs and increases participation.

Communities, the carriers of culture, are important for understanding the social context in which health and illness occur and for determining the most effective interventions. Unlike populations, communities are not concrete or defined by external parameters such as political boundaries or disease categories. Rather, they are subjective. A description of the same community may vary from group to group or individual to individual. The same residentially based population, for example, could be described as a single community by a local politician or as two communities by teachers working in its two school districts or as several communities by members of various ethnic subpopulations. Geopolitically based health departments are most effective when they combine epidemiological and statistical data on populations with an understanding of the cultural matrix of health and illness in the communities they serve and the cultural capital available to address it.

COMMUNITY PRACTICE GOALS

Ultimately, the goal of public health practice is a healthy community. But what is a healthy community? The measure of a community's health is not simply the aggregate of the health status of its individual citizens. Nor is the measure of a community's health found in its most affluent neighborhoods. Rather, it is found in its poorest areas, where unsafe housing, dangerous streets, substandard schools, underemployment, lack of access, and lack of voice are symptoms of social and economic ills that ultimately affect the whole community. A healthy community is a physical, economic, and cultural infrastructure that has the potential to fulfill the overarching goals of Healthy People 2020.

In clinical practice, nurses are responsible for working directly with their patients and families to manage personal health problems. In public health, an essential community health nursing responsibility is enhancing the community's capacity to create a healthy community agenda and to protect and promote the health of citizens now and in the future. Community capacity is the strength and ability of local groups and institutions to manage the various changes, difficulties, and opportunities that will occur over the decades. Although many situations and trends are not within their control, the healthiest communities have a plan for mobilizing material and social resources to manage adverse events and protect the growth and sustainability of community life. (Simmons, Reynolds, & Swinburn, 2011)

In some respects, building community capacity is not unlike helping individuals and families acquire the skills and resilience to successfully manage the problems, losses, crises, and adjustments that occur over a lifetime. In community practice, however, nurses build capacity by identifying and mobilizing community cultural capital and working through and with community leaders, institutions, and groups to create a healthy community agenda for achieving a sustainable future. In places where there is an active citizen infrastructure with a demonstrated capacity for community development and social planning, residents have the best chance for reaching a satisfactory resolution of health and social problems.

To better understand community cultural capital, consider a scenario in which the vision and hearing status of children between the ages of 10 and 14 is to be screened. It is neither necessary nor practical to send each child to an audiologist or optician to be properly assessed. Nor would it be particularly effective to announce the availability of a screening program and just hope that parents and children would show up. Instead, the program can be designed and organized through the school system, where most children are conveniently gathered at predictable times. In addition, school records can be used to identify those children who are absent and require follow-up in order to ensure the evaluation of the entire targeted population. Because schools are part of the community's cultural capital, such programs can be scheduled routinely each year so that every child's performance can be traced over time at regular intervals. Finally, through community action at the policy level, such programs could be funded and budgeted as part of an ongoing responsibility shared by the school systems and the public health department to monitor the vision and hearing status of children annually.

Although this example of schools as cultural capital may seem exceptionally obvious, it is important to understand that each community has distinct characteristics that must be systematically and comprehensively identified and analyzed, incorporated into an inventory of community cultural capital, and mobilized, as necessary, through culture specific action. Thus, parent-child community health practice is not just about providing personal health services in the form of pre-natal care to a target population of high-risk mothers in pre-natal clinics. Rather, it is about identifying community resources available to meet the needs of child-

<table>
<tr><td>

Suggested Activity

Identify three examples of cultural capital in your community.

</td><td>

bearing families in the community—currently and in the future. As discussed in Chapter 1, the community is greater than the sum of its parts and offers more opportunities for intervention than any single member could provide.

</td></tr>
</table>

COMMUNITY ASSESSMENT

Just as clinical practice begins with a systematic assessment of the individual client, community health nursing begins and continues to be informed by a comprehensive analysis of the community client and its health issues, concerns, strengths, and expectations (American Nurses Association, 2007). On entering the examining room, the clinician's first view of the patient includes head, torso, and extremities. Community health nurses, on entering a neighborhood, town, city, or county, may see major highways, a commercial center, schools, factories, government buildings, parks, perhaps a mountain range or prairie, a river dividing commercial areas, a residential suburb, recreational areas, and urban centers easing into farmland.

Whereas the clinician interviews the patient, determining his or her age, ethnicity, residence, religion, occupation, and educational level, the community health nurse determines the socio-demographic characteristics of the population—age distribution, educational level, religions, occupations, ethnic groups, and so on. And whereas clinicians explore the bodily and behavioral aspects of their patients and how they function, community health nurses evaluate the community's social and economic institutions, class structures, neighborhood associations and government, and the ways in which *they* function, alone and with each other, in a specific environment. In direct patient care, health status and health deviations are identified objectively through techniques such as physical examinations and laboratory tests, and subjectively by taking a history and ascertaining the client's perspective on his or her health problem. Both objective and subjective findings are included in the analysis and diagnosis. In community health practice, inferences are drawn from demographic, sociological, environmental, and economic data, as well as from health status and health utilization data. Assessment tools include reviews of biostatistics, epidemiological studies, socio-demographic surveys, and ethnographic research, which may include community based and household studies. In addition to statistical information, community data include local definitions, how community members are related, and the prevailing values related to health and illness. These can be obtained directly by talking with community members and attending community events, as well as from the media, including radio, television, and local newspapers, and from observations of public behavior and community life.

When populations and communities are the primary units of nursing intervention, it is common to think in terms of rates, patterns, and trends when describing actual and potential health problems. For example, an individual patient either has or does not have heart disease, but a population has a *rate* of heart disease that may compare favorably or unfavorably with the rate of heart disease in another population in the community or with a previous time period for the same population. In clinical practice a woman is either pregnant or not, but in community health nursing, it is possible for a community to be "a little bit" pregnant or "a lot" pregnant. Paired with descriptive data about the community, statistical population data are the direct observations and "lab results" that help to diagnose the health of populations and determine a community's health risks. An analysis of the dynamic and synergistic interplay of the environment, the population, and the social organization reveals the cultural capital as well as the health risks of a community and provides the basis for designing a healthy community agenda.

COMMUNITY PLANNING AND INTERVENTION

Clinicians work with patients to determine the health care goals and treatment strategies that make up a care plan. Similarly, public health nurses—in partnership with the community—use assessment data to identify and prioritize the health risk profile of the community and the cultural capital that informs a healthy community agenda. But unlike a patient care plan, comprehensive planning for the community's health is not something that is undertaken and completed within a specific health event, beginning with assessment and ending in evaluation. In fact, the timing and sequencing of public health practice is one of its most distinctive features. Community health nursing is necessarily future-oriented; designing and implementing a healthy community agenda *now* will build its capacity to manage what may occur in 5, 10, or even 20 years.

Things happen more slowly in community health nursing. Compared with direct patient care, in which laboratory tests can be performed, reported, and acted upon in a matter of minutes or even seconds, it often takes months, years, or decades to detect changes and trends in the health status of a community. An education program for teenage parents, for example, may not demonstrate a community wide improvement in early-school performance of their children for three to five years after the program is conceived and initiated. On the other hand, effectively designed community programs such as those in community preparedness may quickly address and evaluate the emergency management of the after-effects of a community disaster. In public health practice, assessment, planning, intervention, and evaluation are ongoing, routine activities required to trace patterns of health, illness, and socio-demographic change in a community. The five- and 10-year plans, revised annually through ongoing assessment, guide and organize the daily, weekly, and monthly activities of community health practice.

By monitoring changes in the ethnic structure of the community's culture, we will be able to predict, for example, the following:

- In the next five years, the number of children under the age of 10 will increase dramatically.

- Many of those children will come from families in which English is a second language.

- A substantial proportion of those children will be in need of daycare while their mothers are in the labor force.

- Much of the care for children with health problems will be carried out by teachers and school nurses.

- Neighborhoods with the greatest influx of children may have safety and health hazards that will affect child welfare and development.

This awareness of trends and the dynamic cultural matrix of the community is essential to anticipate, assess, plan, and prepare for emerging health issues, prevent health problems, promote health, and, critically important, build the cultural capacity to do so.

The future and long range orientation of community health practice poses some interesting dilemmas because the real measure of effectiveness is not how well problems are handled as they occur, but how successfully health is promoted and problems are averted. It is difficult to evaluate the effectiveness of community health nursing because it often is measured by events that, if correctly addressed, will not hap-

Suggested Activity

Compare and contrast the public health management of a rising incidence of environmentally associated neoplastic disease with the clinical management.

pen. In addition, it is not always easy to engage community enthusiasm for results that may not occur for several months or even years. On the other hand, the magnitude of the results in terms of the hundreds, thousands, and even millions of people affected by public health interventions are thrilling and deeply gratifying for those fascinated by the opportunity to build sustainable communities, reshape health care, and ameliorate large-scale health problems.

Personal health services include a well-known range of nursing procedures that are the stock and trade of the clinician. Counseling a parent, changing a dressing, putting a patient through range-of-motion exercises, irrigating a catheter, or teaching a family member how to administer insulin are common procedures in the provision of direct patient care. Community health nursing intervention strategies, on the other hand, include public speaking, journalistic writing, social marketing, record keeping, statistical analyses, program development and evaluation, coalition building and political action, and policy formulation. Interventions take place at the system level and might include promoting legislation to mandate exercise in school, being interviewed on a Spanish-language radio program, writing a guest column on how to select a nursing home, mobilizing support for the cleanup of toxic waste, or analyzing data on sexually transmitted infections (STIs) in a specific community.

For example, several objectives in both Healthy People 2010 and Healthy People 2020 focus on the reduction of asthma, which is one of the top 10 reasons for emergency department visits by children in the United States. Twenty-three million people in the United States have asthma (Bloom, Cohen, & Freeman, 2008), generating annual health care expenditures of $20.7 billion (NIH, NHLBI, 2009).

While deaths from asthma have decreased since the mid-1990s, the prevalence of asthma has continued to increase since 1980, particularly in low-income and minority populations including women and children, African Americans, Puerto Ricans, and employees with workplace exposure. The care plan for a patient with asthma is likely to include breathing and relaxation exercises, inhalation therapy, one-to-one teaching, family counseling, and an emergency action plan. In contrast, the care plan for a community in which asthma is prevalent is likely to include identification of at-risk populations, implementation of screening programs, utilization of media resources for health education, smoking-cessation programs in schools and workplaces, public policy regulating air-pollution levels and smoke-free environments, and organization of community action groups to lobby for control of industrial wastes.

Clinicians and community health nurses may use similar interventions, such as education, but apply them differently. For example, peri-operative nurses provide individualized post-surgical instructions so the patient is informed of what to expect, what to do, where to go, and whom to ask for help in the event of an emergency. This education relieves anxiety, encourages rehabilitation, prevents complications, hastens recovery, and engages the patient in a therapeutic plan of care. Community health nurses, accountable for community wide disaster preparedness, also use education as an intervention to ensure that residents and groups are aware of the disaster plan. To do this, they identify and deploy cultural capital such as schools, radio and television stations, the Chamber of Commerce, and local grocery stores in planning and disseminating the plan, establishing periodic disaster drills, enlisting and educating volunteers, establishing a website, and working with local merchants to stock a "disaster pack" of food, water, batteries, candles, etc.

COMMUNITY COORDINATION

An important responsibility of clinicians is to coordinate the services of other providers such as the physician, social worker, radiologist, physical therapist, and lab technician to increase efficiency and reduce the potential for error in patient care. In community health practice, partners from education, law enforcement, transportation, social services, and housing join public health in identifying, integrating, and deploying resources from every dimension of the community to promote the health of the public. This might include bringing religious leaders of different denominations together with major industries to develop child-health and daycare programs for working parents. Similarly, legislators, industrial leaders, and emission experts could be convened to create policies that will improve the air quality of communities. Community nurses collaborate with local organizations, media resources, and influential community leaders to create healthy communities. The Federal Interagency Workgroup (FIW), which led the Healthy People 2020 initiative, included not only the U.S. Department of Health and Human Service Agencies but also seven other federal agencies representing agriculture, education, housing and urban development, justice, interior, veterans affairs, and the environment.

COMMUNITY EVALUATION

In clinical practice, we evaluate our care to determine how successful we were in achieving the outcomes established by the client and the provider team. This could include recovering from an illness, becoming alcohol-free, reducing emergency department visits for a child with asthma, having an uncomplicated birth experience, or having a peaceful and meaningful death. Efficiency and cost enter the evaluation process in determining whether the same outcomes can be achieved at less cost or whether better outcomes can be achieved at the same cost. In community practice, the desired outcome is the extent to which cultural capital is used to achieve a healthier community—a place that is safer, cleaner, and more tolerant—where people live longer, more productive, and happier lives, and where health equity has been achieved. In community health, evaluation is ongoing and interwoven with assessment, planning, and implementation.

THE NURSE-COMMUNITY RELATIONSHIP

Community health nursing intervention is fundamentally a relationship-building exercise. Trusted alliances with community members and groups are essential for building community capacity and translating resources into a healthy community agenda. The process of engagement includes an openness to and integration of the diverse perspectives of community members.

The comparisons presented thus far suggest compelling differences in the nurse-client relationship in community health practice. Unlike clinical practice, in which nurses see a relatively select category of patients (usually under very private circumstances), public health nurses develop ongoing, sustainable relationships and work with the whole population in everyday community life. It is important for community health nurses to be highly visible, taking part in community events and making themselves known to all sectors of the community and their leaders. Through their reputation and relationships, they cultivate support for public health programs and policy reform.

Although all nurses, consciously or unconsciously, are role models for their clients, role modeling is particularly important for community health nurses. Constantly under the scrutiny of community residents, community nurses exemplify, in appearance and behavior, the expectations they set for community residents. How can community health nurses launch a campaign to eliminate cigarette-smoking in all public places if they are smokers themselves? How do community health nurses convince high-school administrators to initiate nutrition-education programs if they are overweight and have poor dietary habits? And how do community health nurses encourage citizens to vote and engage in public service unless they, themselves, are active participants in community public life?

There is also the critical matter of confidentiality. Therapeutic relationships, grounded in trust and mutual respect, are essential for effective intervention in every nursing situation, whether in clinical or in public practice. It is, however, more complicated in community intervention, where the focus of practice is an entire community of people—some of whom may be at odds with one another or, at the very least, curious and cautious about one another. The betrayal of confidence with just one resident or community organization can generate a community wide lack of trust and easily compromise acceptance and effectiveness of both the public health nurse and associated programs and activities. Maintaining confidentiality, abstaining from judgment, facilitating openness to diverse perspectives of community members, and developing an informed understanding of the culture of the community are essential skills for the practice of public health nursing.

Unlike individual clients, communities are composed of many individuals and diverse groups who may have competing problems and conflicting goals and priorities. To be a potent force in achieving the public's health requires setting aside personal or group loyalties and working for the benefit of the community as a whole. Desired outcomes are achieved through coordination and articulation of community constituents and through win-win strategies. To do this, we must know the various groups and factions of the community, all of which must have—and know that they have—equal access to and the consideration of their community health nurse.

COMMUNITY NURSING VALUES

The fact that communities are composed of groups with conflicting goals and competing values creates unique ethical issues in public health practice. Indeed, one of the most distinguishing features of community health nursing is its value orientation, in which the common good takes precedence over the good of the individual (American Nurses Association, 2007). The public health nurse who provides both personal health services and community level intervention often is caught in a web of competing values. This tension between the individual and society in ensuring the public's health has always existed. Ruth Freeman, a founding leader in community health nursing education in the United States, addressed this explicitly in 1963:

> The selection of those to be served ... must rest on the comparative impact on community health rather than solely on the needs of the individual or family being served. ... The community health nurse cannot elect to care for a small number of people intensely while ignoring the needs of many others. She [sic] must be concerned with the community as a whole. (p. 35)

This passage leaves no room for doubt. Grounded in utilitarian ethics, when there is conflict between individual goals and community goals, community goals must prevail. Such conflicts typically arise when there is competition for limited health resources.

Consider a community in which a small number of individuals could benefit by the presence of sophisticated cardiac technology in a local hospital. The families of these individuals and their cardiologists may present a strong case for having these procedures available locally. On the other hand, the community may achieve more enduring, less costly, and better outcomes if limited resources were directed toward *prevention* of cardiac disease, such as a community based cardiac-health–education program to instruct all families in the community on the principles of good cardiac health.

There are times when community health nurses may have to select among competing goals, both of which are for the good of the whole. Communities are complex aggregates, and although some values are shared among all residents, groups within the community may disagree about particular issues and events. Therefore, not only are there bound to be occasions of conflict between individual- and community level objectives, but also among different factions within communities.

With these opposing demands, how does one define the common good? The good of the whole community does not necessarily mean the desires of the majority. Imagine, for example, a community in which a particular industry, which happens to be the largest employer of community residents, is engaged in a conflict with the health department and concerned citizens regarding its dangerous waste-disposal practices. If compliance with waste-disposal regulations has economic consequences for employees, such as reductions in workforce or decreased wages, it is likely the offending industry will have many supporters in the conflict while the health department will have only a few, despite its more enduring value of its position for the health of the community. Caring for the health of the public requires not only a shift in the practice paradigm, but also a shift in the values that influence priority-setting and decision-making when faced with the inevitable conflict between individual and public health and among special-interest stakeholders within communities. The way in which community health nursing resources (time, expertise, experience, and influence) are deployed must reflect the whole community now and in the future.

3

STRATEGIES FOR ENTERING AND UNDERSTANDING YOUR COMMUNITY

A comprehensive understanding of the community—its health and its culture—is the foundation for building community capacity to protect and promote the health of the public. *Assessment,* the first of the three core public health functions, is a prerequisite for the other two—*assurance,* and *policy.* This chapter describes how to assess the culture and health of a whole community using strategies from two approaches for collecting, organizing, and analyzing information: epidemiology and anthropology, both of which inform public health practice in different but complementary ways.

CHAPTER 3 OBJECTIVES

- Describe how epidemiology and anthropology inform the assessment of the health and culture of a community.

- Differentiate a community health assessment from community based research.

- Learn the strategies and techniques for collecting, organizing, and analyzing information required for a comprehensive understanding of the community.

- Identify the kinds and sources of information obtained about the community.

KNOWING YOUR COMMUNITY—ITS STRENGTHS, ITS ISSUES, AND ITS PROBLEMS

Public health nurses who have worked with the same community for a long time have institutional memories about the residents, environment, politics, and health of their communities. Having internalized all of this cultural information, their decisions tend to be highly effective but often grounded in experience rather than evidence. To be useful for community decision-makers, we need a documented and comprehensive analysis of the community, its health, and its culture. Although public health nurses are responsible for ongoing community data collection and management, they are not researchers. Their goal is not to develop or test new knowledge but rather to apply the strategies and techniques of scientific investigation to acquire information about the community's strengths and cultural capital as well as its needs, issues, and problems. A culturally informed community health assessment will reveal appropriate and effective ways to intervene and promote the health of the community.

Community assessment is the routine and systematic collection, management, analysis, and preparation of information required for culturally informed, community specific planning and action. In clinical practice, patient interventions ordinarily are preceded by an assessment and followed by an evaluation. In public health, however, the collection and management of community data is an ongoing activity to ensure accurate information will be readily accessible. Ethical, cost-effective, and sustainable community change is possible only in collaboration with community citizens and groups. Conducting a community assessment provides an important opportunity to become acquainted with community residents and build trusting relationships. Although it is impossible to interact directly with every member of the community, it is essential to establish an acquaintance and a presence with all sectors of the community. This includes informal groups such as the regulars at the local coffee shop, members of the Red Hat society, or a mothers' morning playgroup at the recreation center. It also includes community leaders from business, education, law enforcement, and religious institutions, as well as representatives of particular ethnic constituencies. Building relationships with community residents and collecting accurate and useful information are mutually reinforcing activities.

INFORMING PUBLIC HEALTH PRACTICE THROUGH EPIDEMIOLOGY AND BIO-STATISTICS

The primary goal of epidemiology is to determine the causes and risk factors of disease and other health problems by identifying and analyzing their distribution among designated populations. Traditionally, the health of communities was measured almost exclusively by the presence or absence of disease in its population—especially acute, infectious disease. Epidemiology, originally the study of epidemics, has now expanded to include chronic illness and other health and social problems such as crime rates, automobile injuries, substandard housing, high-school graduation rates, and health disparities. One research area of epidemiology is to identify the risk factors (e.g., age, ethnicity, tobacco use, obesity, sex) associated with prevailing public health problems. Based on the outcomes, screening programs are implemented for early detection of these risk factors and early community intervention. Epidemiology also identifies populations known as high-risk groups—that is, groups that are especially vulnerable to specific illnesses. Risk groups can be associated with many kinds of factors, such as biological (breast cancer in women), ethnic (diabetes in some Native American groups), socioeconomic (high rates of asthma in children of families below the poverty level) and occupational (chemical exposure in the workplace). Epidemiological data are usually presented using bio-statistics. Before we discuss the contribution of epidemiology to a community health assessment, a brief summary of bio-statistical measures of population health is useful.

BIO-STATISTICAL MEASURES OF POPULATION HEALTH

Birth, death (mortality), and illness (morbidity) statistics ordinarily are expressed as rates rather than absolute numbers because rates enable comparison of the experience of populations with one another, as well as in different timeframes. Each rate is computed by dividing the number of events in question—for example, death by suicide—occurring during a specific time period by the population at risk for the event during the same time period. The phrase "population at risk" means all those persons who have the potential to experience the health problem in question. For example, because women do not have the potential to contract testicular cancer, they would not be counted among the population at risk for morbidity or mortality for that disease. But because all members of a population have the potential for dying, death rates are calculated using the entire population as the denominator.

CALCULATING RATES

$$\text{RATE} = \frac{\text{The number of specified events during a particular time period}}{\text{The population at risk for the event at midpoint during the time period}} \times 1{,}000,\ 10{,}000,\ 100{,}000$$

The numerator and denominator used to calculate rates must reflect the same population in the same time period, with the numerator being included in the denominator. The number in the denominator is computed by using the population at the midpoint of the specified time period.

Rates are expressed as multiples of 100, 1,000, 10,000, or 100,000. The choice of multiplicative factor depends on the size of the population and the frequency with which the event occurs. The rates should be expressed in a figure that is not so small that it must be expressed in a fraction or so large that it is awkward or unwieldy. For example, the mortality rate of AIDS in the early years of the epidemic in the United States was given as a multiple of 1,000,000, because cases were few at that time. Currently, the rate is expressed per 100,000; this reflects the increase in diagnosed cases over the past 20 years. To express the rate of AIDS for a specific city of 500,000 inhabitants, in which there were five reported cases of AIDS, the morbidity rate would be .01 per 1,000, or .1 per 10,000. Although both calculations express the same thing, and thus could theoretically be used interchangeably, one per 100,000 is the least cumbersome and most broadly applied. Convention also tends to dictate the multiplicative factor. Infant mortality rates, for example, are commonly expressed using 1,000 as the multiplicative factor, while maternal mortality rates, reflecting a less-frequent event, are usually expressed using 10,000. In any case, the multiplicative factor should always be mentioned when reporting the rate.

By looking at the rate rather than the absolute number of occurrences, groups of different sizes may be compared to determine the relative severity of the problem in any population. For most purposes, raw numbers are not useful in a community health assessment because they do not lend themselves to comparison with other communities and populations, and thus their significance is obscured. In other words, it is impossible to know if the number of cases is low or high relative to other communities or if it represents a major departure from previous numbers for that community.

Crude Rates

Crude rates, which have not been adjusted to account for age or other factors, may yield unjustifiable conclusions. For example, it would be misguided to compare the crude death rate in a retirement community with that of a community in which elders represent only 5% of the population.

$$\text{CRUDE DEATH RATE} = \frac{\text{The number of deaths}}{\text{Total population}} \times 100,000$$

To make such a comparison, it would be necessary to adjust for the age factor to produce a standardized rate, called an age-adjusted rate. An age-adjusted rate is calculated by assuming the age distribution in all communities is the same, thus eliminating the confounding factor of age. Because age is the single best predictor of overall mortality and morbidity, the age-adjustment of mortality and morbidity rates is crucial for evaluative purposes (Hebel and McCarter, 2006). There are many different kinds of rates that can be used to describe the health status of a population—for example, age-specific rates (the rate of teenage death), sex-specific rates (the rate of alcoholism among females), or any other possible subgrouping of a larger population. The denominator in these instances is only the number of persons in the specified subgroup.

An understanding of statistical rates and how they are calculated is the first step in assessing the health of a population. In clinical nursing, a client's vital signs provide a gross but immediate and important indication of his or her well-being. In population assessment, the vital signs are health status indicators that include not only mortality and morbidity rates, but also many of the statistics presented in Chapter 4, "Discovering the Culture of Your Community," and Chapter 5, "Determining the Health of Your Community." For example, poverty rates, unemployment rates, and the percentage of the population on public assistance all help to predict the kinds and amount of health problems in any given population. The Centers for Disease Control and Prevention (CDC) has recommended a standard set of health status indicators to be used by each state. It is critical for public health providers to know whether their state has developed this kind of instrument and how to access it.

Selecting the health status indicators that will provide the most relevant information about the health of a community depends largely on the community and the concerns of its residents. For example, using maternal-child health statistics to measure the well-being of a retirement community would not be very useful. Nor would it be helpful to rely as heavily on chronic disease rates to evaluate the health status of a developing country that is more affected by infectious diseases.

Mortality Rates

Mortality rates measure the number and categories of deaths. Whereas crude death rates are based on the entire population, specific mortality rates relate to the number of deaths in various categories such as a particular subgroup of the population (for example, children, an ethnic group) or deaths from specified causes (such as accidents or cancer). It is not unusual for the top three causes of death in a particular community to be consistent with national statistics. In most states, death rates are highest for cardiovascular disease, cancer, and stroke. It is the remaining seven in which most local variation is likely to occur and that provide the most significant information regarding the health status of a particular community.

$$\text{CAUSE SPECIFIC DEATH RATE} = \frac{\text{Total number of deaths from a specified cause}}{\text{Total population}} \times 1{,}000,\ 10{,}000,\ 100{,}000$$

Suggested Activity

Investigate the following:

- What are the age-adjusted rates for the five leading causes of death in your community?
- How do they compare with the rates for the previous 5 and 10 years?
- How do they compare with state and national rates?
- What trends and differences are present, and how can they be explained?

Morbidity Rates

Unlike mortality rates, which are concerned with the numbers and kinds of deaths in a population, morbidity rates are concerned with the occurrence of various diseases or health problems in a population. Thus, the number of people who die from cancer is reflected in the death rate, while the number of people who are diagnosed with cancer is expressed in a morbidity rate.

Morbidity rates are reported in terms of incidence and prevalence. Incidence refers to the number of newly reported cases that occur during a specified period of time. Prevalence, on the other hand, is more of a snapshot approach; it refers to the total number of cases (new and old) that exist in a specified period of time. If, for example, a total of 20 new cases of diabetes in a population of 10,000 were reported during 2004, the incidence rate for that year would be 2 per 1,000. Because those 20 join the ranks of the 180 individuals already diagnosed with diabetes, swelling the total number to 200, the prevalence rate for diabetes in the district would be 20 per 1,000.

Occasionally, one sees reference to an attack rate. This is a subcategory of the incidence rate and refers to a very limited period of time. For example, one might use the attack rate to measure the effects of an outbreak of salmonella poisoning or measles during a specific period.

Incidence and prevalence rates have different uses. Incidence rates are used for the following reasons:

- To determine etiology or causation

- To identify trends in disease occurrence

When the incidence rate rises, we suspect that a new etiological agent is operative or that the etiological factors already known have increased in amount or virulence.

The prevalence rate, on the other hand, is used to plan for health services. It gives a current picture of the total number of people who are alive with the illness at a given point in time.

$$\text{INCIDENCE} = \frac{\text{Number of new cases of a disease or health problem occurring during a specified period of time}}{\text{Population at risk at midpoint in time period}} \times 1{,}000,\ 10{,}000,\ 100{,}000$$

$$\text{PREVALENCE} = \frac{\text{Total number of cases of a disease or health problem occurring during a specified time period}}{\text{Total population at midpoint in time period}} \times 1{,}000,\ 10{,}000,\ 100{,}000$$

Increases in the prevalence rate can reflect an increase in incidence plus duration—that is, there are more cases than usual and/or more successful treatment outcomes that result in more people with the illness surviving for longer periods of time. Thus, decreases in the prevalence rate may be due to death or to the discovery of curative treatments. New treatment methods alone do not influence the prevalence rate unless they are successful in curing the illness.

From the size and composition of the population, it is possible to anticipate both the amount and content of health services needed now and in the future. Morbidity data address health problems even more directly and refines predictions of population health status. Both incidence and prevalence rates are important and useful because they give very different kinds of information about the presence of illness in the community. Unfortunately, they often are difficult to obtain at the local level because they require the population to be surveyed, which is very time-consuming and expensive.

Usually, only incidence rates for reportable infectious diseases such as AIDS, tuberculosis, sexually transmitted infections, and cancer are available for local communities. In addition, when the total population of a community is very small, the health department often will not publish these rates for privacy reasons.

Suggested Activity

Investigate the following:

- What are the incidence and prevalence rates of the five leading causes of death in your community?
- How do they compare with the rates for the previous five and 10 years?
- How do they compare with state and national rates?
- What trends and differences are present, and how can they be explained?
- Which populations are disproportionately affected by infectious disease?

EPIDEMIOLOGICAL STUDIES OF POPULATION HEALTH

Monitoring the incidence rate is critical for identifying etiology and new causal agents. Because the resources for doing this often are not sufficient, there are epidemiological research strategies that correlate suspected risk factors with the occurrence of disease when the population incidence rates are not available. These research approaches are known as case-control or retrospective studies and cohort or prospective studies.

CASE-CONTROL STUDIES

When disease prevalence is low in the population or there are limited funds to investigate, a case-control study, also referred to as a retrospective study, may be conducted. Some of the most commonly accepted risk factors have been implicated as a result of case-control studies, including smoking and lung cancer and family history and breast cancer.

Case-control studies can be carried out in a reasonably short period of time and are the most economical to conduct. In them, two groups of people—one with the disease and one without—are identified. These groups are further subdivided into those that have been exposed to the suspected etiological agent and those that have not. This comparison yields a statistic called an odds ratio (OR), which calculates the odds of having the disease when the suspected factor is present as opposed to absent.

Odds ratios are estimations of a statistic called the relative risk (RR), which can be calculated only when the true incidence rate of a disease is available. The higher the odds ratio or relative risk, the more likely the suspected etiologic factor is causally related to disease incidence. In the case of breast cancer, for example, three factors consistently identified by case-control studies with an odds ratio of greater than 4 are (1) older age, (2) birth in a North American or northern European country, and (3) having a family history (mother and/or sister) of breast cancer (Cuzick, 2003). The latter two factors strongly suggest either a genetic or an environmental etiology and, in fact, a gene for breast cancer has been isolated. Impetus for exploring this genetic line of research was no doubt prompted by the strong association found in many case-control studies that linked breast cancer to family history and country of origin. Other well-publicized risk factors for breast cancer, such as multi-parity, early age at menarche, late age at menopause, and alcohol consumption, have lower relative risk—between 1.1 and 2 (Cuzick, 2003).

Case-Control Study

Suppose 220 women with breast cancer are recruited for a study and are compared with 1,140 women who do not have the disease. The total group is further divided into those who have a sister or mother who has breast cancer (exposure present) and those who do not (exposure absent). Typically, a case-control study is depicted as a 2-by-2 table.

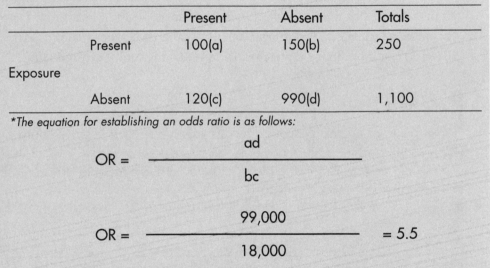

DISEASE

		Present	Absent	Totals
	Present	100(a)	150(b)	250
Exposure				
	Absent	120(c)	990(d)	1,100

*The equation for establishing an odds ratio is as follows:

$$OR = \frac{ad}{bc}$$

$$OR = \frac{99,000}{18,000} = 5.5$$

Thus, the odds of someone with a mother or sister with breast cancer being diagnosed with the same disease in this sample is 5.5 times greater than for someone without a similar family history.

COHORT STUDIES

When sufficient evidence exists to suggest a link between a factor and a disease, a cohort study may be proposed. This type of study, also referred to as longitudinal, examines the disease experience of a cohort of people over time. Cohort studies could be historical, in which case the records of large groups of people exposed to a certain risk (for example, workers in an asbestos manufacturing plant) are examined for past levels of exposure and disease occurrence. They also can be prospective, in which case a total population or representative sample is followed over time, and morbidity and mortality rates are related to study variables.

Much of what is known about risk factors for coronary heart disease comes from an ongoing prospective study begun in Framingham, Massachusetts, USA, in 1949 (National Heart, Lung and Blood Institute and Boston University, 2011). Cohort studies of this type are very useful but often prohibitively expensive. Using the cohort design, a relative risk can be calculated by dividing the incidence rate of a disease among those exposed by the incidence rate among those not exposed. Thus, relative risk measures the strength of the association between a factor and an outcome (Hebel and McCarter, 2006). Again, the higher the odds ratio or relative risk, the more likely the factor being studied is causal or etiological.

Cohort Study

A group of nurses is followed for 40 years, from first licensure until the present, and the occurrence of lung cancer is recorded. A total of 40,000 nurses are enrolled in the study, and they are divided into smokers and nonsmokers.

DISEASE

		Lung Cancer	No Lung Cancer	Total
Risk Factor	Smokers	1,400(a)	14,600(b)	16,000
	Nonsmokers	200(c)	23,800(d)	24,000

The equation for calculating the relative risk is as follows:

$$\text{Relative Risk} = \frac{\text{incidence rate among exposed}}{\text{incidence rate among nonexposed}}$$

Thus, in this case, the equation reads as follows:

$$RR = \frac{a/(a+b)}{c/(c+d)} = \frac{1{,}400/16{,}000}{200/24{,}000} = 10.5$$

In this sample, it can be concluded that the probability of developing lung cancer is 10.5 times higher for nurses who smoke than for those who don't smoke.

Causal relationships are demonstrated even more strongly by calculating the difference in disease occurrence in groups exposed to the factor to different degrees—for example, comparing the odds ratios or relative risks from case-control or cohort studies for lung cancer in those who smoked one, two, and three packs of cigarettes a day. If greater exposure results in a higher odds ratio or relative risk, a dose-response relationship is established, with causality more likely. In fact, this is exactly how the now widely accepted causal relationship between smoking and lung cancer was established.

The rate and kind of illnesses and disabilities that prevail in a community offer a more refined measure of the health of a population than do birth and death rates. Patterns of morbidity are determined and anticipated not only from incidence rates of reportable infectious diseases, but also from prevalence rates of chronic diseases and disability; maternal-child health indices, such as percentages of pregnant women receiving adequate prenatal care; and rates of mental-health and behavioral problems, such as depression, substance abuse, and tobacco-smoking. In the best of all possible worlds, all of this data would be readily available and recorded in a format that would encourage comparability over time, between sub-population groups, and at state, national, and international levels. This is not always the case, however; it is very important to know where and how to access data for a comprehensive community health assessment.

INFORMING PUBLIC HEALTH PRACTICE THROUGH ANTHROPOLOGY AND ETHNOGRAPHY

As described above, epidemiology identifies those groups of people who are at risk for specific health problems through the correlation of health concerns with specific population characteristics. Although such correlations reveal potential risk factors, the exact causes often are difficult to isolate with certainty without additional—often costly—studies. Because the origins of epidemiology are in medicine, it is especially useful for comparing populations according to the biological and physiological characteristics of their component individuals. Socio-cultural determinants, in comparison, are more difficult to manage epidemiologically and often are treated as if they were characteristics of individuals rather than of the environments in which the individuals are located. Thus the influence of culture on childhood asthma is calculated by correlating the incidence or prevalence of asthma with ethnicity, national origin, or language (individual characteristics). Although this may result in a strong association between childhood asthma and ethnicity, we cannot know, without additional studies, whether it is because children of that ethnic group are more likely to live in a congested urban area, are exposed to more cigarette smoke in the home, or some other unknown factors. And even a robust association between ethnicity and childhood asthma provides only limited information to help us determine the best public health action plan.

In comparison, anthropology—using ethnographic methods—provides a broader understanding of the socio-cultural factors that affect health and illness and how they are related. Ethnographic methods typically include long term immersion and participant observation in community life, not unlike community health nursing practice. Ethnography is descriptive and comparative—as opposed to experimental or correlational—and seeks to capture the perspective of the local people. The goal of ethnography in public health is to reveal the community level factors that collectively influence the community's health and the health of its citizens. Using the community rather than individuals aggregated in populations as the unit of analysis, comparison and context analysis are used to explore the sources of both the problems and the solutions—for example, what are the local factors that distinguish neighborhoods with a high rate of childhood asthma from those with a low rate? Additionally, how is childhood asthma linked to the socio-cultural factors of local life? For example, where and when are most asthma emergencies recorded? Which groups of children are likely to be affected? What are the dynamics between childhood asthma and social class or between asthma and social institutions such as education and recreation? Unlike epidemiology, which is focused on identifying at-risk populations, ethnographic descriptions try to identify the cultural matrix in which illness is caused and health is produced.

UNDERSTANDING THE MATRIX OF HEALTH AND ILLNESS THROUGH ETHNOGRAPHY

The ethnographic strategies of anthropology offer useful approaches to public health for identifying culture specific solutions as well as problems. So how do we begin to acquire an understanding of our community's culture? Using ethnographic strategies (Bernard, 2011), our investigation begins with the big picture—the whole community as both the object (the health of a whole community) and the context (the place in which health, illness, and public health intervention occur) (Arensberg, 1961; Drevdahl, 1999). Our inquiry then becomes increasingly issue- and problem-focused. Before we begin working on a particular health issue or problem, whether its low–birth-weight infants, obesity, air pollution, disaster preparedness, or safety for older adults, we need to be grounded in an understanding of the community as the constellation of place, population, and social organization. Then we can begin to analyze and understand specific public health problems in the context of the community in which they occur.

If, for example, epidemiological studies indicated that obesity in preschool-age children in our community is increasing, we would want to find out which families in our community have this problem, where they live, and their ways of life. Are they distributed throughout the community, or are they concentrated in particular neighborhoods or income groups? How do the families of these children intersect with the larger community? Where do they work, where do they recreate, and how do they procure and prepare food? What is different about these families from similar families in which preschool-age children are not obese? Perhaps most importantly, we would want to know what it is like to be a preschool-age child in this community. Who cares for them during the day and prepares their food? What and where do they eat? Where and with whom do they play? Were they breast-fed or bottle-fed? Do they go to daycare or to preschool programs? What amount and kind of physical activity do they get during the day? Gathering information about the community context gives us a better understanding of the source of the problem and enables us to identify the cultural capital that will help communities to address the problem.

GATHERING COMMUNITY DATA

When we conduct a health assessment on an individual patient, we review a combination of laboratory data, patient reports, and provider observations. Similarly, community health assessments combine many kinds of objective and subjective data as well as quantitative and qualitative data, each of which contributes to a comprehensive understanding of the community and a basis for interpretation of health and illness. In community health practice, there are three main sources of data we use in an ethnographic approach for conducting a culturally informed community health assessment:

- What we observe directly about the community

- What people tell us about the community

- What is documented about the community in newspapers, radio and television, historical sources, census reports, vital records and bio-statistical reports, epidemiological surveys, websites, etc.

Suggested Activity

In a personal and confidential Community Practice Notebook, record observations and interactions. Include newspaper clippings, flyers, articles, and other documents collected in the process of entering and learning about your community. These data then will be organized according to the community culture inventory outlined in Chapter 4 to prepare a culturally informed community health assessment.

Community Practice Notebook*

Date: _____

Goals for this community assessment activity: _____

Description of the activity: _____

> Write about and/or draw diagrams to describe the experience you had in the community. Do not judge it or evaluate it. Describe it so that when you read through this at a later time you will have a clear picture and understanding of the experience. If you are doing this correctly, it will take time and thought to complete the entry. This is important because you will use some of this description to complete your culturally informed community health assessment. Include the following:

> - *Professional interpretation:* As you record information about the community, also note your initial interpretation based on the literature that you have read, course work, class discussion, research, practice models, and your thinking about the experience

> - *Personal reactions:* Describe your response to the community and the people you have met. From your perspective, what went well? What didn't go well.

Plans for next community practice activity:

> *Include the following:*

> - *Professional:* Describe areas that you want to assess further, resources or collaborative relationships you will explore, community models, programs and interventions, objectives and goals, effectiveness, and/or modification of the strategic plan.

> - *Personal:* Describe your ideas for how you may handle the situation in the future and resources you will explore for your own growth and understanding.

* This is a personal and confidential notebook but identities of community members in the notebook should be protected in case of loss or theft.

WHAT WE OBSERVE DIRECTLY ABOUT THE COMMUNITY

Before we begin the process of building relationships in our communities, we can learn a great deal simply by touring the community and observing various neighborhoods. Is there, for example, a downtown? Are there topographical features such as rivers and mountains, or human-made environmental features such as superhighways, bridges, or boardwalks that can both separate and unite various components of the community? To have an understanding of the physical community, it is useful to have at least three maps:

- One that outlines the major topographical features of the community (mountain ranges, hills, rivers, lakes and ponds, seashore, etc.)

- One that designates the regional position of the district/community in relation to urban centers and outlines the transportation system in and out of the community

- One that denotes settlement patterns, streets, highways, residential areas, commercial areas, and major institutions such as schools, churches, commercial centers, and official buildings

By posting the vulnerable aspects of the community on these maps (for example, tracts of poor housing, congested streets, personal injury crimes, environmental hazard areas, epidemics, polluted water, and so on) as well as the community strengths (for example, schools, health centers, faith-based institutions, recreation areas, etc.) you create a visual representation of the community's culture.

Suggested Activity

Use Internet mapping tools such as http://earth.google.com, as well as paper and pencil, to sketch out the landmarks as you drive and walk around the community.

Residents' use of time is equally as important as their use of space for understanding both the sources of and the solutions for poor community health. Various populations and institutions of a community have different schedules and cycles of activities. Community celebrations and holidays, along with major religious festivals, school vacations and events, ethnic celebrations, and historical occasions constitute the rhythm of local culture. These time-specific aspects of community life are recorded on a series of schedules and calendars demonstrating daily, weekly, and seasonal variations in community activity. Information about how particular groups in a community use time should include all hours of the day, seven days a week, and all the seasons of the year. Limiting observation to Monday through Friday, nine to five, may fail to capture important aspects of public health, such as criminal activity, traffic-safety issues, and availability of emergency care.

Suggested Activity

Post community events and cycles on an annual calendar. Post patterns of community activities on weekly and monthly schedules.

Attending routine community events such as public hearings, religious services, and parent-teacher association meetings, and visiting shopping centers, school playgrounds, train stations, and movie theaters reveal the culture of local life, group-held values, and how time and space are used by residents and visitors. The goal is to be as comprehensive as possible. Both the calendar/schedules and the various maps are working documents, always being revised and updated. The most useful calendars and maps are likely to look cluttered and a little chaotic. They will, however, provide a useful visual inventory of the community's use of space and time over a year and the implications for public health.

> A family-planning project designed to bring contraception education to rural Caribbean communities included a fully equipped van with an electric generator, a film projector, and a full assemblage of family-planning materials. Family-planning educators were selected, trained, and scheduled to visit several communities each week. The presentations were usually scheduled in the evening, on a weeknight, and were ordinarily filled to capacity. The attendees, however, were mostly older children and men. The women of childbearing age were home looking after their small children. Although it is certainly advantageous for all community residents to be exposed to the concept of family planning, the target population for whom the program was intended was not there. The program planners had neglected to take into consideration that in these rural communities, men are nighttime gatherers while women are daytime gatherers. Had the program been held on Sunday at various churches in the community, in the marketplace on Saturday, or at rural clinics on a weekday, it is likely more women of childbearing age would have been reached.

Before we move on, a few comments about first impressions are in order. Our initial view of communities often changes dramatically once we get to know our places and people. Peace Corps workers reported being overwhelmed by the crowded streets, poorly clothed people, disrepair of the homes, and freely wandering goats and pigs when they first entered what they thought were impoverished communities to which they were assigned. After being in the country for several weeks and exposed to other communities, however, they reclassified their first communities as working class. Best clothes were reserved for religious days, and houses were modest but not in dangerous disrepair. The families in these communities had access to resources including livestock, were sending their children to school, and were making strides toward social and economic improvement in a complex environment. No matter what communities we enter as public health professionals, inferences are subject to observer bias or prejudgment and will change as we come to know more about the community and its culture. It is important, nonetheless, to record first impressions and occasionally return to them. In the process of becoming familiar with a community, one begins to take some of its characteristics for granted. Our first impressions help us understand the reactions of newcomers and to retain objectivity about the community to which we have become accustomed.

WHAT PEOPLE TELL US ABOUT THE COMMUNITY

Meeting and talking with community residents and leaders as you begin the process of building relationships reveals much about the community. It is important to remember, however, that each person's perspective will reflect his or her particular position in the community—for example, length of residence, occupation, neighborhood, age, sex, and socioeconomic status. You should not be surprised, therefore, when different members of the community give very different—even conflicting—reports about the same community issue or event. One person may claim her neighborhood is changing for the worse, while another may describe it as revitalized and an exciting place to live. The greater the number and variety of community residents you meet and talk to, the more complete the picture of the community culture. This includes not only those community members who represent or are affiliated with the health care system, but also those who interact with the public on a routine basis and have a different vision of the community, for example, public officials, religion leaders, teachers, librarians, politicians, merchants, hairstylists, restaurant owners, bartenders, real-estate brokers, bankers, journalists, or police officers.

Focus groups are another means of collecting data that help the nurse understand community health behavior, strengths, and problems. Originating in market-research companies, focus groups are used for gathering the opinions of community members. A focus group is composed of carefully selected individuals—usually between six and 12—who engage in an exploratory discussion of specific topics, sharing their experiences and offering opinions. The discussion is recorded and lasts about 90 minutes. Customarily, these groups are scheduled for at least one additional meeting after the participants have had an opportunity to review the first session, to answer additional questions or confirm the findings of the first session. In addition to providing helpful information regarding a public health issue or problem, focus groups are also a strategy for engaging residents in community improvement. A focus group consisting of adolescents, parents, teachers, coaches, police officers, and insurance executives convened to examine the issue of driving safety among teenagers may also be the kernel of a future community group dedicated to reducing traffic accidents.

Although the reliability of subjective reports from community members is occasionally questioned, it is important to acknowledge that even carefully designed surveys and reports reflect the biases of those being interviewed and those doing the interviewing. Any kind of inquiry captures only the kind of information that individuals and groups are willing to share. Police reports published in local newspapers, for example, do not tell us about the amount and kind of crimes actually committed in a community but rather about the crimes that citizens, police, and newspapers choose to report. Similarly, depending on the reporting organization, population statistics may over- or underestimate the size of an ethnic group. This is why the names and positions of community residents should be recorded as well as their own words and exact opinions. For example:

> *At Central City Town Meeting Mr. Johnson, principal of Central High School, stated that he would not support Representative Snyder in the next election because she opposed the introduction of sex education in the public school system.*

is more useful than writing:

> *Educators from Central H.S. engaged in a lively discussion about sex education and local politics.*

In the first statement, the relationship among education, politics, and sex education is clear, not just from the perspective of any community resident, but from one who holds a pivotal position and works regularly in all three arenas. This more specific statement helps us understand current political issues, draw inferences about local sexual mores, and know who would or would not support programs that address the issue of adolescent sexuality. In assessing a community, it is necessary to know not only what was said or written, but also who said or wrote it.

WHAT IS DOCUMENTED ABOUT THE COMMUNITY

Many communities with access to the Internet have a web page. Although such web pages ordinarily portray the town, city, or county in the best possible light, they are still useful for acquiring an understanding of self-identified community strengths and are a good starting point for your inquiry.

Two additional documents that provide a good introduction to the community's culture are the phone book and newspapers (including small, advertisement-based papers). If the community does not have a newspaper of its own, the closest local newspaper will at least reveal the way in which the community is perceived regionally. The *Yellow Pages* of the telephone directory list hospitals, churches, recreational facilities, schools, daycare centers, physicians, lawyers, businesses, and other services for residents that are useful in an inventory of community resources and cultural capital.

There are many other formal sources of community information, including the local library, Chamber of Commerce, government offices, department of educa-tion, police and fire departments, and parks and recreation offices. City- or coun-ty-planning commissions, if they exist, are particularly valuable. A benefit of per-sonally visiting local organizations is the opportunity to meet the most knowl-edgeable members of the community, inform them of the community health assessment, and obtain the most up-to-date information sources. Finally, a good source of socio-demographic data is the most recent census (http://www.census.gov/; http://factfinder2.census.gov/main.html).

A problem in using documents prepared by various community organizations is that they often are in units that are not coterminous with each other or with your designated community. Information pertaining to children may have been com-piled by school districts, data on communicable disease may have been compiled according to health districts, and data on public sanitation and safety may have been compiled according to fire and water districts or police districts. This is par-ticularly true in more complex urban environments, where public institutions and offices have divided up the state, county, or city pie in different ways. Not only are these various districts not coterminous, they may cut across census tracks as well as community boundaries. The use of the data will require some judgment and an acknowledgement that some data is better than no data. The relative value of some sources of information over others is simply a function of their use- fulness in addressing the question being asked.

For example, if the public health topic being addressed is the nutritional status of schoolchildren, there are several approaches to understanding the problem:

- We could ask children to complete a questionnaire on their 24-hour nutritional intake.

- We could review the school menus over the past three months and evaluate the nutritional content of the meals.

- We could rely on direct observations of eating behavior and food consumption by schoolchildren during mealtimes.

Each of these kinds of information has advantages and disadvantages. In the 24-hour nutritional intake, the children may consciously or unconsciously report wholesome food consumption and neglect to mention the candy bar or potato chips purchased from a vending machine. School menus provide reliable informa- tion on what was served, but not on what was actually eaten. Direct observa- tions, in this case, are probably the most revealing source of information but are very expensive to collect because you cannot observe all the children at the same time. The most complete and easily obtained picture of the problem is derived from a combination of the three sources of information.

For some kinds of public health issues, direct observations may not be the best source of information. For example, if we were formulating a five-year plan for the provision of prenatal services in a specific community, observations and inter- views with childbearing women in prenatal clinics may be much less useful than census reports and data on migration patterns, economic changes, and birth and infant statistics over the past decade. Different sources of data also permit the examination of both values and behaviors and the discrepancies that often exist between what people say when asked or surveyed and what people do in real life. For example, community members might report that they value good health and believe cigarette-smoking is bad, yet observations may reveal that they continue to smoke. Teachers might instruct children in the principles of good nutrition in the classroom but raise no objections to the installation of a candy vending machine in the school cafeteria to increase school revenues. Identifying discrepancies and conflicts between what people say and what people do is critical knowledge for designing community health action plans that work.

Again, no matter which sources of data are included for the community assessment, it is always more helpful to report specific behavior and events than general impressions. In clinical practice, the information recorded in the patient's chart is expected to be exactly what is observed and heard. The same expectation applies to public health. For instance, reporting that:

> *Last year, there were 22 incidents of assault and robbery in which the victim was 75 years or older, in comparison with 5 years earlier, when there were none.*

is more revealing and more powerful than saying:

> *Victimization of elders is a growing problem in this community.*

Specific information citing the growing incidence of crimes against older adult citizens helps to make a better argument for securing resources such as transit service for those over 75 years old or increasing police surveillance for older citizens. In addition to recording community observations and conversation, it is important to critically review the information in documents. Every type of information has inherent strengths, biases, and limitations that are important to acknowledge when designing a culturally informed community health assessment. Similar to the information that comes from what people tell us, documented and published information also reflects the perspective of the people and organizations who wrote and published them and the purpose for which they were to be used. Local newspapers, for example, will necessarily reflect the political and philosophical biases of the editors. Material assembled by the Chamber of Commerce will attempt to cast the community in a positive light to attract businesses. Information collected by the health department, on the other hand, may be oriented more to community health concerns, health promotion, and disease prevention.

ACCESSING PUBLIC HEALTH DATA

Though information about the culture and health of a community is not always formatted to immediately answer the public health questions we may have, all levels of government are charged with collecting data about various aspects of community life, ranging from education to economic status to health. With the advances of electronic communication, we have more data than at any point of time in history

THE UNITED STATES CENSUS

Mandated by the U.S. Constitution in 1790, the census is conducted every 10 years. Socio-demographic information, including various aspects of health and social life, are collected, analyzed, and reported for the entire United States and subdivided into states, counties, cities, towns, and census tracts.

Conducting the national census is an enormous undertaking. Although it's true that the census data are less current by the time they are analyzed and reported, the census remains very useful for showing trends over time and establishing a national database for benchmarking progress. The census data are extrapolated from a weighted representative sample. Some of the census statistics must be defined before interpretation. The unemployment rate, for example, can be subject to a wide range of definitions. The census also makes an important distinction between families and households, which is highly useful for community health purposes. Most of the census data are available on the Internet and in libraries. In addition, most states have a databank center that produces a condensed summary of each geopolitical unit (that is, town, city, and county).

THE CENTERS FOR DISEASE CONTROL AND PREVENTION (CDC)

Located in Atlanta, Georgia, the mission of the CDC, an agency of the U.S. Department of Health and Human Services, is to promote health and quality of life by preventing and controlling disease, injury, and disability. The CDC is responsible for gathering information on all reportable diseases, collecting data from state health departments, and conducting and sponsoring research on various health problems in the United States. The *Morbidity and Mortality Weekly Report* (MMWR) published by the CDC summarizes information on common infectious diseases on a national level and contains news on specific outbreaks of diseases in various areas of the country. A most recent example is the CDC publication of the "HIV/AIDS Surveillance Report." Similar data are available on the international level from the World Health Organization (WHO).

The National Health Survey, first conducted in 1956, contains synthesized information about the state of health and health services in the United States. Using probability-sampling techniques, ongoing surveys of households permit estimates of the prevalence of specific health problems, including minor illnesses and disability. Since then, many surveys have been developed that constitute ongoing national data sets—for example, the National Health and Nutrition Examination Survey (NHANES), which measures the general health status of the total U.S. population, and HHANES, which measures the health status of Hispanic Americans.

STATE HEALTH DEPARTMENTS

State health departments usually are a good source of relevant health data and reveal county-by-county differences in health status. They vary, however, in their requirements for reporting disease and the extent to which residents are surveyed for specific health problems. These data are particularly useful if health services are organized on a county basis. For example, in some states, records are kept on all firearms-related injuries treated in all emergency rooms. Other states may have the capacity to provide health status indicators to local communities. Although most libraries have a government-documents department to facilitate access to these statistics, increasingly data are available through the Internet or through computer programs developed specifically for these purposes.

LOCAL SOURCES

Birth and death registries (which also are organized by the federal government) and state, municipal, and county records on mortality and morbidity statistics are sources of current data. Schools and industry ordinarily keep records on group absenteeism, accidents, injuries, and other health problems. Many record group results of personality inventories, intelligence tests, and various screening programs, as well as utilization data such as immunization programs, counseling and education centers, and visits to the school nurse.

Records from hospitals, clinics, and other health agencies, including professional associations and health care voluntary associations, are yet another source of local information on population health. Unlike school and industry records, they reflect only utilization data rather than health status data. They do not take into account all those who have a health problem (incidence and prevalence data), but only those who are receiving care. Because many people who are in need of health care do not access it for various reasons, utilization statistics fall short in accurately describing the level of morbidity and predicting the need for health services. Information derived from all health provider agencies, therefore, must be supplemented with data from other sources to acquire the most comprehensive picture of the health status of a community. Local health departments may have data based on a recent assessment of health needs as a basis for local planning efforts, and thus are the repository of much useful information about the health problems of a community and resources available to deal with them. The county coroner's office can be helpful in gathering data on deaths by accident, suicide, and homicide.

HEALTH SURVEYS AND EPIDEMIOLOGICAL STUDIES

National, state, and local health surveys provide even more detailed and equally important sources of data about the occurrence, distribution, and causes of current health problems. These surveys are undertaken routinely by the government, schools, hospitals, voluntary associations such as the American Cancer Society and the American Heart Association, and universities engaged in epidemiological or health policy research. Together, these surveys provide longitudinal and cross-sectional data on the population's health.

Although sources vary in the degree to which the information is accurate and reliable, dated or less-comprehensive information should not be dismissed. It may be the only information available. Using imperfect information simply requires that it be identified as such and interpreted with caution. Because judgments of poorer or better community health status rely on comparisons with other communities; with state, national, and international statistics and indicators; and with other time periods, a wide range of sources must be accessed. Federal agencies that are sources of national health data sets list Internet links to state departments of health. The following section lists credible Internet sites that provide not only comprehensive data, but also quick snapshots of health statistics at international, national, and state levels. Many of these sites derive from the World Health Organization (WHO) and the Centers for Disease Control and Prevention (CDC), which house the global and national health statistics, respectively.

INTERNET SOURCES FOR HEALTH STATISTICS

Listed in the next sections are helpful resources for public health work. This is a mere sampling of the resources available.

Suggested Activity

Using Web-search tactics, identify additional information on the area in which you are working or researching.

International Health Resources

■ AIDS Information Global Information System (http://www.aegis.com)

■ International Agency for Research on Cancer (http://www.iarc.fr)

■ International Association of Gerontology and Geriatrics (http://www.iagg.info)

■ Joint United Nations Programme on HIV/AIDS
(http://www.unaids.org/en/default.asp)

■ World Health Organization (http://www.who.int/en)

■ World Health Organization, Ageing Topics
(http://www.who.int/topics/ageing/en)

U.S. National and Governmental Health Resources

■ Agency for Healthcare Research and Quality, U.S. Department of Health and
Human Services (http://www.ahrq.gov)

■ American Nurses Association, Government Affairs
(http://www.nursingworld.org/gova)

■ American Public Health Association (http://www.apha.org)

■ Centers for Disease Control and Prevention, U.S. Department of Health and
Human Services (http://www.cdc.gov)

■ Centers for Disease Control and Prevention, U.S. Department of Health and
Human Services, *Morbidity and Mortality Weekly Report*
(http://www.cdc.gov/mmwr)

■ Centers for Disease Control and Prevention, U.S. Department of Health and
Human Services, Diseases and Conditions
(http://www.cdc.gov/DiseasesConditions/)

■ Centers for Disease Control and Prevention, U.S. Department of Health and
Human Services, National Center for Health Statistics
(http://www.cdc.gov/nchs)

- Centers for Medicare and Medicaid Services, U.S. Department of Health and Human Services (http://www.cms.hhs.gov)

- ChildStats (http://www.childstats.gov)

- Federal Emergency Management Agency (http://www.fema.gov)

- HealthFinder, National Health Information Center, U.S. Department of Health and Human Services (http://www.healthfinder.gov)

- Healthy People 2020 (http://www.healthypeople.gov)

- Medicare (http://www.medicare.gov)

- National Cancer Institute, U.S. National Institutes of Health (http://www.cancer.gov)

- National Consumer Protection Week (http://www.ncpw.gov/about-us)

- National Institutes of Health, U.S. Department of Health and Human Services (http://www.nih.gov)

- Office of Minority Health, U.S. Department of Health and Human Services (http://www.omhrc.gov)

- Public Health Foundation (http://www.phf.org)

- PubMed, U.S. National Library of Medicine and National Institutes of Health (http://www.ncbi.nlm.nih.gov/pubmed)

- The Congressional Institute (http://www.conginst.org)

- Trust for America's Health (http://healthyamericans.org)

- U.S. Census Bureau (http://www.census.gov)

- U.S. Census Bureau, American FactFinder (http://factfinder.census.gov/home/saff/main.html)

- U.S. Census Bureau, New American FactFinder
  (http://factfinder2.census.gov/main.html)

- U.S. Department of Health and Human Services (http://www.hhs.gov)

- U.S. Food and Drug Administration (http://www.fda.gov)

- U.S. Food and Drug Administration, Center for Food Safety and Applied
  Nutrition (http://www.cfsan.fda.gov)

- U.S. White House (http://www.whitehouse.gov)

U.S. State-Based Resources

- Ask SPHERE (Southeast Public Health Educational Resource for Enhancement) (http://www.asksphere.org)

- Commonwealth of Massachusetts Health and Human Services
  (http://mass.gov/dph)

- Iowa Department of Public Health
  (http://www.idph.state.ia.us/chnahip/reports.asp)

- New England Alliance for Public Health Workforce Development
  (http://sph.bu.edu/otlt/alliance)

- Pacific Public Health Training Consortium, Web Links
  (http://www.pphtc.org/resources/onlineresources.htm)

Environmental Resources

- Earthlife Web (http://www.earthlife.net/index.html)

- Environmental Law Net (http://www.lawvianet.com)

- Scorecard (http://www.scorecard.org)

- United Nations Environment Programme (http://www.unep.org)

- U.S. Environmental Protection Agency (http://www.epa.gov)

- U.S. Environmental Protection Agency, Envirofacts Data Warehouse (http://www.epa.gov/enviro/html/qmr.html)

- U.S. Environmental Protection Agency, Office of Air and Radiation (http://www.epa.gov/oar)

- U.S. Environmental Protection Agency, Superfund (http://www.epa.gov/superfund)

- U.S. Environmental Protection Agency, Superfund, Waste and Cleanup Risk Assessment (http://www.epa.gov/oswer/riskassessment/index.htm)

- U.S. Environmental Protection Agency, Water (http://www.epa.gov/ebtpages/water.html)

- World Resources Institute (http://www.wri.org)

- World Wildlife Fund's Global Environmental Conservation Organization (http://www.panda.org)

Population Resources
- The Population Institute (www.populationinstitute.org)

- Population Reference Bureau (http://www.prb.org)

- United Nations Population Fund (http://www.unfpa.org)

Topic-Specific Resources
- Administration on Aging (http://www.aoa.gov)

- American Cancer Society (http://www.cancer.org)

- The John A. Hartford Foundation (http://www.jhartfound.org)

- Medscape (http://www.medscape.com)

- National Breast Cancer Coalition (http://www.natlbcc.org)

- OncoLink (http://www.oncolink.upenn.edu)

- Y-Me National Breast Cancer Organization (http://www.y-me.org)

PULLING IT TOGETHER: CULTURALLY INFORMED COMMUNITY HEALTH ANALYSIS

In community practice, collecting and analyzing community information are not only ongoing and systematic, but often intertwined. The Culturally Informed Community Health Assessment Tool is a useful reminder of the range of information that usually is needed. It provides an outline for capturing information about the community's culture and health, and then categorizing that information so that inferences can be drawn. This process makes it possible to draw comparisons within the community, as well as with state, regional, national, and international populations. It also permits comparisons to be made regarding previous time periods, so current trends and the shifting patterns in community life can be understood.

Culturally Informed Community Health Assessment Tool
Community Culture Inquiry

I. Physical Environment of a Community
   A. Spatial dimensions
      1. Boundaries, size, and distribution
      2. Regional position
      3. Geophysical and climate factors
      4. Land use
      5. Housing
      6. Transportation
      7. Communication
      8. Mental maps
   B. Temporal (yearly, monthly, weekly, daily working calendars and schedules)
      1. Community history
      2. Cyclical population movement
      3. Economic cycles

    4. Psychological cycles

    5. Cyclical crises

II. Population of a Community

  A. Total population (size, density, distribution)

  B. Temporary subpopulations

  C. Biological composition (age and sex)

  D. Ethnic and racial groups

  E. Occupation, income and education level

  F. Residential and household characteristics

III. Social Organization of a Community

  A. Community institutions

    1. Economic

    2. Government, politics, and law enforcement

    3. Domestic

    4. Religion

    5. Education

    6. Recreation

    7. Voluntary

B. Horizontal stratification

C. Vertical segmentation

Community Health Assessment

I. Environmental Health

  A. Outdoor air quality

  B. Surface- and ground-water quality

  C. Food contamination

  D. Toxic substances and hazardous-waste management

       1. Solid waste

       2. Sewage

       3. Radioactive waste

       4. Chemicals and pesticides

    E. Noise pollution

    F. Disease vectors

    G. Preparedness

    H. Crime

    I. Accidents

    J. Homes and communities

    K. Community buildings

    L. Energy management

    M. Global health

II. Population Health

    A. Infectious diseases

    B. Chronic diseases

    C. Chronic disability

    D. Behavioral and Mental health

    E. Maternal, infant, and child health

    F. Early and middle childhood health

    G. Adolescent health

    H. Older adult health

    I. Lesbian, gay, bisexual, and transgender health

    J. Occupational safety and health

    K. Population health behaviors

III. Health Care Organization: Institutional and Ideological Dimensions

    A. Health Workforce such as:

       1. Nursing

       2. Medical

   3. Dental
   4. Social work
   5. Mental Health
   6. Nutrition
   7. Optical/Audiology
   8. Therapies, such as Physical, Occupational, Speech
B. Public Health Agencies
   1. Health Departments
   2. Personal Health Care Agencies such as
      a. Hospitals ("health centers")
      b. Nursing homes, extended care facilities, assisted living
      c. Home health agencies
      d. Freestanding ambulatory facilities
   3. Health Planning Agencies
C. Public Health Financing
   1. Third Party Payers
      a.   Commercial
      b.   Government
   2. Self-pay
   3. Charity
   4. Public Assistance
D. Health Values and Beliefs
   1   Customs
   2. Traditions
   3. Values
E. Indigenous and Alternative Health Systems

An ethnographic exploration of the community culture provides the context in which health risks and problems, identified through epidemiological studies, are interpreted, prioritized, addressed, and ameliorated. Illnesses, injuries, safety problems, and unhealthy behaviors are better understood by examining them in the socio-cultural milieu, where they occur and interact. High rates of cancer, for example, could be related to the presence of a nuclear energy plant and faulty methods of waste disposal in one community, while in another it could be linked to the age distribution of the population. Both communities have a high rate of cancer, but plans for effective prevention, advocacy, and system level intervention must vary according to local conditions and cultural capital.

The community culture inquiry (discussed in Chapter 4) and the community health assessment (discussed in Chapter 5) have descriptive and analytic components that provide a culturally informed picture of the community's health, health risks, and cultural capital. In public health practice, there are four basic questions that need to be asked of all the information acquired in our community culture inquiry and health assessment:

- How does the community information vary with time? For example:

- In the culture inquiry: How does the number and quality of housing units compare with the previous five or 10 years?

- In the health assessment: How does the current incidence of elder abuse and neglect compare with the previous five and 10 years?

- How does the community information compare with similar communities and with local, state, national, and international findings? For example:

- In the culture inquiry: How does the proportion of residents over 65 compare with the proportion of those individuals at the state, national, and international levels?

- In the health assessment: How does the community's rate of Alzheimer's and other dementias compare at the county, state, national, and international levels?

- How does the information in the various categories of the culturally informed community assessment relate to information in other categories? For example:

- In the culture inquiry: How are community programs serving older adults related to politics or economic factors?

- In the health assessment: How are disparities in elder services linked to time, place, population characteristics, and social organization?

- What are the implications of the community information for health and health care? For example:

- In the culture inquiry: What are the implications of a tourist-based economy for the health of elder community residents?

- In the health assessment: What effect would alcohol use by middle-age adults have on the elder population in the community?

4

DISCOVERING THE CULTURE OF YOUR COMMUNITY

Culture is not just about ethnicity. Rather, it is about the way in which a community uses space and time, its life ways, and the manner in which people are organized and interact. It also includes the way in which health is promoted, illness is prevented, and care is provided. From a systematic examination of the community's culture, we begin to identify issues and problems. Perhaps even more important, we discover its strengths—the cultural capital for achieving the goals of Healthy People 2020. This chapter offers a protocol for gathering, organizing, and interpreting information about the culture of a community.

CHAPTER 4 OBJECTIVES

- Learn a systematic and comprehensive procedure for gathering and recording the environment, population, and social organization of a community.

- Develop strategies for identifying the community's strengths, issues, and concerns.

- Use comparison and contextual analysis to determine the impact of community culture on health and illness.

COMMUNITY CULTURE INQUIRY

The assessment and analysis of community culture presented in this chapter follow a protocol that was developed by Conrad Arensburg (1954, 1955, 1961) and Solon Kimball (Arensberg and Kimball, 1965) to facilitate the application of anthropology in community development and social services. It approaches the study of communities through three different but related aspects of culture:

- Its physical environment

- Its population

- Its social organization

Within each of these three large components of community culture are subcomponents that provide greater detail for understanding a community.

This culture inquiry is not intended to be exhaustive, but rather to provide a simple and meaningful way to organize community culture information into categories so that comparisons can be made and inferences drawn. The most important goal is not to complete every category and subcategory, but rather to learn an orderly, systematic way of learning about the community and managing the information so that it is most useful.

This holistic examination of the community's culture uses strategies that are not unlike the ethnographic methods used by anthropologists when they enter a culture unknown to them. Although the strategies may be similar, the goals of the community health nurse and the ethnographic researcher are quite different. The researcher is interested in developing new knowledge that will help explain the relationship of human behavior to health and illness. The goal of the community health nurse is a comprehensive understanding of community culture to build the community's capacity for better health. This includes the identification of cultural capital that can be deployed to mobilize community action. It also includes discovering features of the community that may at first appear to be unrelated to health and illness, but in fact are highly consequential for constructing and implementing a culture based healthy community agenda.

THE PHYSICAL ENVIRONMENT OF A COMMUNITY

The physical environment or place of a community includes both the space and the time it occupies. The spatial aspect of a community refers to its natural dimensions (hills, rivers, forests, oceans) as well as its human-made environment (highways, buildings, bridges, street plans). Together, these comprise the setting (rural county, urban neighborhood, or coastal village) in which populations work and live (Eberhardt and Pamuk, 2004; Bender, Clune & Guruge, 2007). In addition to space, the physical environment of a community occupies time. Communities have both a history and a future that influence what can be accomplished in the present. They outlive individual members and successive generations, ranging from infants to seniors, and reflect an orderly progression of the population through days, seasons, and years. The community's history and future ambitions are just as much a part of community life as its rivers, roads, and buildings.

SPATIAL DIMENSIONS OF COMMUNITY LIFE

Communities occupy and use space and its contents in different ways and are shaped accordingly. For example, many of the cities in the northeastern United States that were settled in the last century were built around a waterfall to power the textile or paper mills on which their economies were based. The typical settlement pattern in such communities consisted of worker houses built on flat ground, while the owners and high-level managers lived in more elegant accommodations in the hills. Examples of this type of settlement can be found in communities throughout New England. Midwestern agricultural communities, in comparison, were settled in family-dominated clusters of houses located in a more egalitarian manner, along roads leading to the town's "main street" commercial and service centers.

The spatial aspect of community life is a good place to initiate a community examination because it does not necessitate extensive interviews or interactions with residents. With direct observation, reference to maps, and drawing community diagrams, much can be learned about the community, its health problems, and its resources. Community practitioners working in remote areas of less technologically developed communities may need to create their own maps indicating major topographical features and social institutions. Most communities, however, have fairly detailed maps that can be obtained from the Internet, local planning departments, or municipal or county offices.

Population Boundaries, Size, and Distribution

Suggested Activity

Do the following:

- Obtain a street map of the community.
- Tour the community and draw a map of the space, including natural and human-made features.
- Identify the physical boundaries of the community.
- Record the size of the community in square miles.

Community practice begins with knowing where the unit of service delivery begins and ends. It is therefore necessary to start by identifying the physical boundaries and the size, expressed in square miles, of the geo-political territory to be served. Depending not only on the size of its population but also the way in which it is distributed, it could be geographically small, such as a city block, or it could encompass several rural counties. The physical size of the community in square miles will strongly influence community practice. Responsibility for a large population in a few city blocks is likely to be very different from, but equally as demanding as, responsibility for a small population scattered over many square miles.

Regional Position

Suggested Activity

Acquire a map that demonstrates the regional position of the community. Then do the following:

- If it is a service center, designate the services available to surrounding communities.
- If it is a satellite, designate where community residents obtain various services.
- Designate commuting relationships between the community and other communities, such as work, kinship, and leisure activities.
- Determine the distance, in time and miles, to the nearest urban center.
- Determine how the community relates to the geopolitical units in which it is located.
- Determine whether the community is a town, county, borough, village, or part of a municipality.

The regional position of a community indicates how it is situated in relation to other communities—whether it is a satellite to a larger city or other municipality, or a center to which smaller communities are linked on a daily basis. The degree to which it is isolated from surrounding communities will influence both the strengths and problems of a community. For example, in a community that is remote, the public health nurse may need to emphasize self-help programs, such as first-aid readiness and health literacy. On the other hand, there are advantages to working in communities where kinship and neighbor networks can be mobilized more easily.

The regional position of the community is significant because many problems cannot be resolved at the local level. People may live in community A, for example, but are getting sick where they work, in community B. Individuals who travel daily from the suburbs to the city and back again not only are commuters, they also are carriers of health and illness from one location to another. In addition to work ties, strong social ties often exist between members of communities that are widely separated geographically. For example, many Puerto Rican families living in New York City send their children to Puerto Rico during summer vacations to stay with grandparents. It would be difficult to understand the culture of the specific neighborhoods in New York City without consideration of the family's ties in Puerto Rico. Similarly, it is not unusual for Mexican men residing in the Midwest with their families to return to Mexico routinely to check on their relatives and secure less-expensive health care.

Geophysical and Climate Factors

Suggested Activity

Do the following:

- Identify the natural features of the environment that serve as an organizing force in the district/community (rivers, mountains, plains, coast).
- Identify the human-made features of the environment that serve as quasi-organic forces (superhighways, high-rise apartment complexes, industrial parks, bridges, tunnels).
- Record the climatic conditions of the area (precipitation, winds, temperature range).

The geophysical and climatic features of the community, such as mountains, rivers, or coastline, may be organizing forces in community life. Construction sites are common features of the landscape on urban island settlements such as Hong Kong, Singapore, and Manhattan, where older buildings are continuously razed and replaced by newer, taller ones. In contrast, cities such as Los Angeles and Dallas sprawl indefinitely into their environments. Although some geophysical and climate features, such as mudslides, floods, forest fires, and earthquakes, impose various threats on the health of a community, others provide opportunities for recreation and community gatherings. Human-made physical features such as multi-lane highways, bridges, tunnels, and clusters of high-rise buildings or industrial parks serve as semi-organic forms that affect the health of communities and human activity. A superhighway, uniting several communities, makes it possible to centralize social and economic activities, providing support for a healthy community agenda. At the same time, it may physically divide previously connected neighborhoods and impose several health hazards such as traffic accidents, air pollution, and harmful noise levels.

Land Use

Suggested Activity

Outline the functional designations of land in the community: residential, recreational, commercial, industrial, agricultural, official, and spiritual or religious use. Describe the patterns of land use by the population:

- Areas open to all members
- Areas open to specific community members (old, young, women, ethnic groups).

Communities create various kinds of boundaries. Some have settlement patterns where sections of the community are designated for a special function, such as residential, commercial, industrial, governmental, spiritual, or recreational. In other communities, residents sleep, eat, work, play, and worship within the range of a few blocks; there is no geographical separation of various community activities. The designation of different locations for different community functions generates patterns of assembly and dispersal of community residents. Gathering points such as commercial centers or industrial complexes may bring community members together for certain periods of the day or week, while scattered residences take them in separate directions for the remainder of the time. It is important to identify areas of assembly where many residents can be reached at the same time. In some communities, the most efficient way to reach larger numbers of adults might be through their place of employment, while in others it may be at religious services or shopping centers.

Communities may be organized according to the special characteristics of the residents, such as ethnicity (Little Italy or China Town), or by class (the "ghettos" or Peacock Hills), or even by occupation, such as enclaves of artists and musicians or university faculty. These cultural specifications of territory within communities often highlight health disparities. In addition, many communities have been and continue to be characterized by segregation (Azevedo-Garcia, Lochner, Osypuk, and Subramanian, 2003)—one of the principal reasons for the movement to desegregate school districts. Specific groups may informally designate a particular area of the community as their own "turf" and create boundaries that are not visible to the outsider, but are well-known and well-respected by local residents.

Local conventions governing who may go where in a community have implications for health planning and intervention. An example of this was a lead-screening program held at a fast-food restaurant on a Saturday. A favorite gathering spot for young families on the weekend, the restaurant was considered an ideal site for reaching preschool-age children. In terms of the number of children screened, it was extremely successful. In terms of reaching the population most at risk, however, the program failed. No one had taken into consideration that the lower-income families in which children were most likely to have lead exposure would be unlikely to bring their children to a fast-food restaurant located out of their own neighborhood. A better understanding of the use of space by people in the community and how different groups have different access to space could easily have averted the problem and saved the necessary expense of an additional program.

Housing

Suggested Activity

Do the following:

- Acquire pictures of the range of housing types in the community.
- Map the types of housing on the street map.
- List the number of housing units by single family, multiple family, high-rise apartment building.
- Describe the type of structures.
- Describe access to gardens, lawns, and parks.
- Record types of housing materials, such as wood frame, cement, brick, thatch, mud, cardboard box, or tent.
- Record the age and condition of housing.
- List utilities available in dwellings (for example, water, lighting, cooking facilities, heat, and waste disposal).
- Record household facilities, including furnishings, appliances, and communication devices.

Housing plays an important role in providing a safe, healthy, comfortable, and aesthetically pleasing context for individual and family growth. In addition to providing shelter for a population, it is directly related to the quality of family relationships and to both the psychological and physical dimensions of health. The type of construction and the placement of housing units in relation to each other and to community gathering points influence the ways in which residents interact. Apartment buildings in which there is a common courtyard, swimming pool, or laundry area, for example, are likely to foster more interaction among building residents than a high-rise, dormitory-like building where one rarely sees the person who lives in the apartment next door. Many cities, such as Chicago, have replaced high-rise dwellings with three-story, townhouse-type housing for this reason.

Access to a piece of land for gardens or recreation is another important feature of housing. Many innovative urban planners have transformed vacant lots into vegetable gardens, subdivided and tended by apartment-dwellers. In addition to solving the aesthetic and safety problems that accompany vacant lots, such gardens provide city residents with the opportunity to produce, preserve, and perhaps even sell fresh food. Such community gardens also can become a focal point for community activity, such as outdoor markets, bringing urban residents together.

Housing must be examined in relation to the characteristics of the people residing in the community. It may be very difficult for immigrants who were living in adobe, single-story homes with a detached kitchen to adjust to the high-rise housing of urban centers. Housing units that were constructed for one group, such as young families, may not work as well for elders who require elevators, wheelchair ramps, and perhaps different kinds of lighting. Much of modern housing is electricity-dependent and subject to energy crises in summer or winter months, creating a potentially serious problem for older adults. Finally, abandoned housing has generated a widespread community safety problem, attracting gang members, illicit drug users, and homeless urban squatters.

Transportation

Suggested Activity

Do the following:

- Obtain transit maps of buses, subways, ferries, and waterways. Include a list of the costs of transportation.
- Map patterns of spatial movement within and between residences, workplaces, commercial centers, and schools.
- Outline major arteries, available routes, and public and private transportation.
- Describe the transportation links between the community and the nearest urban centers.
- List the radio stations that serve the community.

> List the television stations and those that provide public health programs.
>
> Identify Internet connections and the presence of social media.
>
> Map out social marketing, such as billboard advertising.

The designation of different zones for different community functions and events requires a transportation system to move people from one activity to another. In addition to knowing how land is used in the community, it also is necessary to understand the way in which people use the network of roads, waterways, and other public transportation.

> When a hospital in a large city decided to close its pediatric clinic, a nearby hospital began to plan for the influx of families it assumed would be drawn from the closed service. It was the closest hospital by distance; however, the journey required a transfer from one bus line to another. Most mothers found it more convenient to go to another clinic that was actually farther away but could be reached on one bus line, without the inconvenience of a transfer.

Communication

The communication system is a critical capacity building tool. Radio, television, newspapers, and the Internet link individuals and groups both within and outside the community for health education, disaster preparedness, and public participation in health planning and policy. Health editors of local newspapers and hosts of local television and radio health programs are important resources for disseminating information about health and for ensuring the participation of community residents in health issues. Several nurses have initiated newspaper columns and television and radio programs to bring health information to the public. Internet services and social media have expanded the capacity for public communication (although they also may simultaneously pose a danger through increased access of pedophiles and other predators). Finally, despite the advantage of electronic media, print media cannot be discounted: Health officials in a very ethnically diverse city found the most effective and efficient way to reach its multicultural population was through several well-read ethnic newspapers that translated the information into the language of its readers.

Mental Maps

The famous cartoon depicting a New Yorker's perspective of the United States, which, looking west, includes first New Jersey and then the West Coast with nothing in between except Chicago, is an example of a mental map. Persons living in Missouri, Montana, or Alabama are likely to have very different but perhaps equally distorted mental images of the United States. Community residents also may have a view of their surroundings that departs greatly from the actual geography. For several years, social scientists have used mental maps (including drawings by residents of their community) to discover the interface of the psychological topography with the physical topography. In doing so, they have identified invisible peaks of psychological stress that residents are afraid to enter, and valleys of safety where they feel comfortable and unafraid.

The names and nicknames applied to certain neighborhoods and sections of the community also tell much about how various neighborhoods are viewed. It is not unusual, for instance, for recently gentrified neighborhoods to have two names: one that is used by the residents who were born and grew up in the neighborhood and another that is used by the wealthier newcomers. This use of two names to describe the same place is telling. It may mirror social and economic differences between the two types of residents and suggest not only how various residents perceive themselves, but also how they perceive the others. It alerts us that there might be a need to use a different strategy for community action with each category of resident.

As with the "turf" aspects described earlier, sacred areas, areas of fear or safety, and other psychological features are superimposed on the physical features. Often, they are not demarcated, and they may go unnoticed by the newcomer to the community. Sensitivity to mental maps is important, however, for understanding the perception people have of their environment and ensuring access to health care services for all populations in a community.

Suggested Activity

Do the following:

- Record sections of the community distinguished by the residents themselves, and what names or nicknames are applied to them.
- Map the areas of the community that frequently are avoided or identified as unsafe.
- Map areas of the community that are designated as sacred or historical, such as ancient burial grounds and memorial parks.

TEMPORAL DIMENSIONS OF COMMUNITY LIFE

Every community has daily, weekly, monthly, seasonal, annual, and multi-annual cycles of activities that comprise the cultural use of time. These temporal factors are especially important in community health practice because timeliness is often a critical factor for successful capacity building. If immunization programs are offered at a time when they are inaccessible to community residents, the participation rate will be low. Public health issues requiring legislative action are likely to get the most visibility and candidate support close to elections.

Community History

Suggested Activity

Do the following:

- Draw a historical timeline of the community.
- Record the date and circumstances surrounding the settlement of the community.
- Describe patterns of population growth since the community was first settled, including waves of migration.

- List the milestone events in the history of the community, including both natural and human-made events—for example, economic changes; wars; major social events; community accomplishments; opening of new roads, railroads or bridges; and disasters.
- Obtain a historical map of the community and designate the place and time of major physical alterations.
- Designate changes in community settlement patterns, such as a shift from downtown to suburban and then back to downtown, on the time line.
- Designate major economic trends in the community on the timeline.
- Designate major political trends on the timeline.

The community of today is largely a result of its history. Specific events and trends have worked to shape the place and its people. Knowledge of the history of the community is important for tracing and interpreting patterns of health problems over time and predicting those that will occur in the future. Understanding the local history is essential for strengthening a healthy community agenda by framing it in local traditions. Historical details of the community are not as important as a general knowledge of what has made the community what it is. There already may be a history written about the community, either because it has a particularly interesting history or because it was done as part of a community event or celebration. If there is no history available in the library or official archives of the municipality or county, there are other sources of history ordinarily available, such as interviews with older residents, newspaper series, public records, census reports, school records, directories, deeds and old maps, and church records.

Cyclical Population Movement

Suggested Activity

Do the following:

- On daily and weekly schedules, identify routine community activities.
- On an annual calendar, record community events that take place each year.
- Identify seasonal changes in the community.
- Record how community use of time varies with various segments of the population.

To plan and implement public health action, it is very important to know the daily, weekly, seasonal, annual, and biannual changes in the population. The movement of people from one place to another generally takes place with a degree of regularity and needs to be included in the community assessment to ensure the health and safety of community residents. For example, to ensure the safety of children coming and going to school, it is necessary to know when automobile traffic is heaviest and when children are most at risk.

Seasonal changes in the population often include major shifts in population, such as tourists and college-student workers who expand the population in the summer months on Cape Cod or double the population of Amherst, Massachusetts, from September to May. These seasonal fluctuations in population size have profound public health implications. The tourists who populate the New England ocean resort towns and "snowbird" migrations of retired adults to Florida in the winter months present resource challenges for creating a safe environment that range from water rescue to sanitation to restaurant inspection to traffic safety.

Economic Cycles

This category of the community inventory includes temporal variations in the local economic structure, including cyclical variations in productivity, employment, occupation, income, and expenditures. The influence of seasonal variation in the local economy on health and health care is apparent in agricultural communities. In communities where agricultural sugarcane production is the main economic activity, for example, hundreds of workers are employed during a six-month period, both in the field to cut the cane and in the factory to process it into sugar. During this time, cash is in the greatest circulation, and people have the resources to pay off their debts and make new purchases. It is also the time when utilization of health care services increases dramatically, often taking care of problems that have been deferred during the leaner months. Additionally, seasonal work patterns and industries, such as agriculture and construction, have high rates of traumatic deaths (Healthy People 2020), requiring public health safety intervention.

Suggested Activity

Do the following:

- Record weekly, monthly, and seasonal work patterns such as regular periods of unemployment, cycles of productivity, and seasonal occupational changes.
- Record periodic changes in income and expenditures.

Psychological Cycles

Suggested Activity

Do the following:

- Chart the psychological cycles of the community:
  - Periods of euphoria and dysphoria
  - Festivities and holidays
- Chart leisure and recreation periods in the community.
- Identify periods of widespread melancholy.

Communities have periodic cycles when either psychological elevation or depression is generalized throughout the population. In most American communities, holidays and other times of ceremonial activity are seen as periods when there is a great deal of anticipation and enthusiasm, with opportunities to be with family and renew old friendships. It also is the time period with the greatest incidence of suicide. Often, euphoric seasons are followed by dysphoric periods when the excitement of the holidays is over, work has resumed, bills must be paid, and weather keeps people indoors and isolated from friends and recreational activity. The first warm days then bring a return of euphoria, with the anticipation of spring and summer and the resumption of social interaction and physical activity.

Student health centers report similar patterns. Each semester begins with the excitement of new classes and new friends. Then as the semester wears on, students are faced with assignments, tests, and papers to be completed, and a fairly predictable midterm dysphoria sets in. At that point, it is common to hear students say they cannot wait for the semester to be over and even express doubt as to whether they will be able to complete their course of study. During these periods of stress, absenteeism is most likely to occur, comparatively minor complaints take on an enhanced significance, and visits to health services increase. At the same time, faculty members feel equally stressed—perhaps in response to students—creating a system wide emotional decline. In comparison, during periods of euphoria, it is not uncommon to hear students say, "I don't have time to get sick; I'm getting ready to go home for the holidays," or "I'm not going to miss homecoming just because I have the flu." During these periods, complaints are minimized and health service utilization decreases.

Cyclical Crises

Suggested Activity
Do the following:
- Chart recurring crises on an annual calendar/schedule.
- List the sporadic crises that have occurred over the past 20 years

Practically all communities have crises that recur on a fairly predictable schedule. Spring flooding, annual flu epidemics, hurricane season, and winter fires are common examples of critical events that take place more or less regularly. According to Healthy People 2020, drowning, the second leading cause of injury-related death in children and adolescents, is a seasonal event. Because seasonal events are relatively predictable, public health measures can be instituted to attempt to either prevent such events or minimize the damage that will accompany them.

Nurse midwives practicing in a remote and mountainous community reported bringing pregnant women across the river each year before the rainy season, when the normally shallow and easily fordable river began to swell. This is an example of anticipating problems and finding ways to ameliorate them or soften their impact.

For example, presenting a prevention program on summer safety, including water safety and first aid, at the end of the school year could both reduce the number of events over the summer and equip children to provide assistance. Hurricanes, tornadoes, forest fires, seasonal floods, and other seasonal disasters require an educated citizenry that knows what to do to help others minimize the impact of a disaster.

In addition to the seasonal crises, there are other disasters that have the potential to occur. Fires, tornadoes, tsunamis, earthquakes, major epidemics, mining disasters, nuclear disasters, and now, of course, terrorist attacks all require preparation. The goal is to develop and maintain the community's capacity for readiness to reduce the impact by having a community plan in place. In a healthy community, the potential for such crises is identified, and a plan is in place for an inter-professional team including health- and human-service professionals such as sanitation and safety engineers, police, communications networks, and rescue teams.

THE POPULATION OF A COMMUNITY

An examination of a community's culture must include a review of its actors—the people who live and work in the community. The number of people in a community and their attributes will influence the capacity of a community to create a healthy future. The population can be examined as a whole, in terms of its size, growth, and distribution. It also can be examined in terms of the bio-cultural and socioeconomic characteristics of its members. These characteristics tell us much about the kinds of public health problems that can be anticipated; they also provide information about the strengths of the population and facilitating a healthy-community agenda. As we learned from our examination of the community as a place, the population of a community is not necessarily stable. Additionally, depending on how it is defined, it may include residents who spend only part of the year or part of the week in the community, or even those who come there every day but return to another community at night.

Population Size, Density, and Distribution

Suggested Activity

Do the following:

- Record the size of the population of the community.
- Identify weekly changes in the population.
- Identify seasonal changes in the population.
- Describe the density of the population (that is, people per square mile).
- Map the distribution of the population between urban and rural areas.
- Chart the changes in the size of the population over the past 20 years.

An understanding of the population begins with knowing not only how many people reside in the community, but also how the population is distributed. Rural localities have been highlighted in Healthy People 2020 as one of the six factors accounting for the nation's health disparities. Defined as communities with fewer than 2,500 residents, rural residents comprise 25% of the American population. Some health related needs are unique to rural conditions and lifestyle (Healthy People 2020). At the same time, we know that many urban neighborhoods also have unique public health issues, ranging from street safety and gang violence to the absence of grocery stores and fresh produce.

Depending on the size of the community, it may have both urban and rural sections and areas of high and low density. In addition to current size and density, changes in the population create new public health concerns. Population assessment begins with an accounting of trends over the past several years, including patterns of migration—both to and from the community—and natural increases or decreases, determined by birth and death rates.

Temporary Subpopulations

Suggested Activity

Do the following:

- Identify the persons who enter the community on a daily basis but who do not live there.
- Identify the persons who stay in the community on a weekly basis.
- Record the seasonal subpopulations residing in the community:
    - Tourists
    - Military
    - Seasonal workers
    - Students

Some communities have special groups, such as the military, summer residents, students, migrant workers, or other groups who may reside in the community but are not of the community. In some instances, such groups may contribute to the economy of the community and have positive attributes that enhance the cultural capital of the community. On the other hand, they may strain community resources, compromising community capacity for health. In any case, the presence of these groups must be accounted for in ensuring the future health of the community. This includes identifying their numbers, major characteristics, roles within the community, strengths, prevailing health risks and problems, and the resources they can offer to build community capacity for health.

Biological Composition: Age and Sex

Suggested Activity

Do the following:

- Record the median age of the population.
- List the percentages of the population from 0 to 5, 6 to 14, 15 to 19, 20 to 34, 35 to 49, 50 to 64, 65 and over, 65 to 74, 75 to 84, and 85 and over.
- Compute the dependency ratio of the population.
- Identify the sex composition of the population.
- Identify the sex ratio of the population.
- Compute the age/sex quotient of the population.

When providing direct care to individual patients, it is necessary to know their biological characteristics to make accurate nursing diagnoses and formulate appropriate care plans. The same principle holds true when providing care to an entire community. The age and sex distribution of a population tells us much about the kinds of health concerns that residents of the community are likely to experience now and in the future, as well as their impact on the health of the community. Age and sex are, perhaps, the most fundamental of the biological characteristics, because so many community health problems are linked to gender and stage of development. For example, the aging of populations and reduction in communicable diseases throughout the United States has mandated an expansion of the emphasis from child health and infectious diseases to managing the health of the chronically ill and elder community residents.

In statistical compilations, the age of a population is presented as the percentage of the population that falls into proscribed categories. The utility of age categories, however, depends on the community. For example, if a setting has a large proportion of older adult citizens, the "over 65" group might be subdivided into "young elders," age 65 to 74; "mid-elders," age 75 to 84; and "frail elders," age

85 and over. At the same time, two of the adult categories might be collapsed into one large group from 35 to 64, simply because the community doesn't have large numbers of individuals in those particular age groups. In other words, the categories should be refined in a way that reflect and are most useful for the particular community.

The proportion of the population under 15 and over 64 is computed as the dependency ratio, meaning it is the part of the total population that is considered to be economically and socially dependent on the rest of the population. It also is the proportion of the population that is likely to require the most health resources. It is therefore a significant figure for public health consideration.

Men and women differ in the kinds of health problems they experience and the manner and frequency with which they use health services. Acknowledging that some sex-specific health problems are biologically based, Healthy People 2020 highlights gender as one of the five categories in which health disparities must be addressed, while also emphasizing that the longer life expectancy in females cannot be attributed solely to biological factors (National Center for Health Statistics, 2011). The sex ratio of a community helps us to understand and predict prevailing health concerns and the need for resources. As the sex that bears children and generally lives longer, it is not surprising that women use more health services than men do. Furthermore, health problems that were once attributable primarily to the male population, such as cardiovascular disease, now are emerging with increasing frequency among females. A high sex ratio—that is, a predominance of either males or females—signals a need to review community services for men, women, and children.

Once the age and sex composition of the community has been determined, it is useful to cross tabulate these two factors to determine the sex ratio within each age category. This greater refinement of age and sex data permits even more predictability as each age group moves to the next developmental stage. For example, it is usually assumed the 65-and-older category is predominantly female, but a closer investigation of the community may reveal that military service and migration have left particular communities lacking in males in one age group and increasing their proportion in another. For example, for several years, the older adult population in Chinese communities in many U.S. cities was predominantly male, reflecting the wave of Chinese immigrant men who came to the United States in the first half of the 20th century as laborers. As each age group moves through its next developmental sequence, its sex composition will have an impact on the health of the community and the necessary health services.

Ethnic and Racial Groups

Suggested Activity

Do the following:

- List the various ethnic/racial groups found in the community.
- Calculate each ethnic/racial group's percentage of the total population.
- Record the percentage of the population that identifies itself as multiracial.
- Determine how homogeneous or diverse the various racial and ethnic groups are.

Race and ethnicity constitute another of the factors highlighted by Healthy People 2020 that are linked to health disparities in this country. According to the U.S. Census Bureau, approximately one-third of the U.S. population belongs to a racial- or ethnic-minority population (U.S. Census Bureau, 2008a; 2008b). Ethnicity and race are two distinct categories that often are misapplied (Drevdahl, Phillips, and Taylor, 2006; Phillips and Drevdahl, 2003; Wolf, 1994). Ethnicity is the complex of traits that identify a group of people based on characteristics such as common ancestry, language, and/or religion. Race, on the other hand, is a more controversial concept. Although we commonly think of race as a biological attribute based on a person's phenotype and genotype, contemporary social science conceptualizes race as a socially constructed category. In the United States, for example, a person whose appearance (or phenotype) is "White" is considered "Black" if his mother happens to be African American. "Hispanic" is a common racial category on health and census surveys, implying, incorrectly, that people of Spanish origin constitute a separate racial group from white or black.

Neither race nor ethnicity can be determined from an individual's phenotype or genotype. Because census reports and health surveys, however, often use categories that group people according to White, Black, or Hispanic, it is important to have a basic understanding of how race is used in public health. With the geographical clustering of populations and a resultant common gene pool, it is not uncommon for specific health problems to have a genetic origin and thus appear with greater frequency in some groups than in others. It is well-known, for example, that sickle-cell anemia is found more often in African-American and Caribbean-American populations, Tay-Sachs disease in some Jewish groups, skin cancer in those of northern-European ancestry, and diabetes in American Indian groups. Certain groups also have inherited resistance to specific diseases. Cancer, for instance, is comparatively low in American Indian populations. Thus, at the community level, race and ethnicity can inform the identification of risk for problems likely to require public health action such as screening and health education.

Many health problems correlated with particular ethnic groups are not caused by an inherited predisposition, but rather from the social position, socio-economic status, or conditions of employment of particular groups or subgroups. The combination of biological and social factors can result in variable health status. For example, the higher rate of hypertension in some African-American and other groups has been related to the stress associated with a lifetime of discrimination (Dressler, 2004). Race and ethnicity have a profound influence on the health and sustainability of communities. They can be the source of community conflict, isolation, uneven distribution of resources, poor health, and ultimately health disparities. On the other hand, as cultural capital, they may be a source of strength and richness in mobilizing and uniting communities.

Prejudice and discrimination have not been confined to groups of color, as the history of the Irish and Eastern European Jews in 19th- and early-20th-century America attests. In cases where discrimination has been legally sanctioned, however such as with African-American populations until the 1950s, the quality and quantity of prejudice has been particularly deplorable. For example, well into the

20th century, laws prohibited African Americans from patronizing many restaurants, hotels, health care facilities, and educational institutions. The unique circumstances of African-American populations must be acknowledged to appreciate the vast differences in opportunity that have characterized various ethnic and racial groups over time (Carlson and Chamberlain, 2004).

Suggested Activity

On the Healthy People 2020 home page, compare the leading cause of death among the different ethnic and racial populations.

Occupation, Income, and Education Level

Suggested Activity

Do the following:

- Record the per capita income in the community.
- Record the mean and median family income and household income.
- Record the percentage of the population with income below poverty level.
- Record the percentage of the population receiving public assistance.
- Record the unemployment rate by age and sex.
- Identify the percentage of females in the workforce.
- List the major occupational categories of the population—for example, professionals, technical workers, managers, officials, proprietors, craftsmen, artisans, operatives, farmers, laborers, domestic workers, etc.
- Determine the percentage of the population over 25 that has completed high school.
- Determine the percentage of the population over 25 that has completed college.

Income, occupation, and education influence many aspects of health and health care. There is no question that populations with high rates of unemployment, poverty, and public assistance will be subject to more public health problems (Rodwin and Neuberg, 2005; Szwarcwald, Dorrea da Mota, Damacena, and Pereira, 2011; Webb, Simpson, and Hairston, 2011). Generally, the problems in poorer communities are more complex because the resources to resolve them are less accessible. According to the Secretary's Advisory Committee on National Health Promotion and Disease Prevention Objectives for 2020, inequality in income is highlighted as a key social and physical environmental health determinant underlying health disparities (Healthy People 2020).

Interpreting the impact of occupation and income requires evaluating indicators, such as average income per household, within the local economic context. For example, an average family income of $50,000 per year may be more than sufficient to meet the household needs of families living in some rural areas of the United States but totally inadequate for a similar family residing in Southern California or Boston, Massachusetts. Differences in economic profile are associated with other differences, such as age distribution or ethnicity. Evaluating the income level of a population must be done in relation to the cost of living within the same region.

In addition to the income level, the occupational composition of the population affects the health of a community. For example, mining and textile manufacturing pose high public health risks for respiratory problems. The proportion of adult females in the workforce signals the need to determine the effects of employment and occupation on women's health, including fertility. It also raises the question of whether there are a sufficient number of high-quality daycare centers for the young children of working mothers. Finally, mothers' education levels are a universal predictor of child health and development worldwide. Because a large component of public health intervention is educational, the educational status of women in the community is an important indicator. Education, similar to income, requires evaluation in relation to the context. In some communities, a high-school education is meaningful and will be the standard even for the community's most prominent citizens. In other communities, it may represent the most minimal preparation.

Residential and Household Characteristics

Suggested Activity

Do the following:

- Record the percentage of the population over 16 that is currently single, married, divorced, and widowed.
- Determine the number of family units in the community.
- Determine the average population per household.
- Record the percentage of single-person households in the community.
- Record the number of owner-occupied households.
- Record the number of tenant-occupied households.
- Record the percentage of the population living in substandard housing.

Different kinds of household configurations distinguish neighborhoods and communities. The prevailing domestic units may consist of young singles or old singles, single parents and their children, grandparents and grandchildren, or any number of combinations, as well as the conventional nuclear family. Because the household generally is the unit of personal health care, it is important to know how many households are in the district. A population of 3,000 divided into 500 households will create very different public health considerations than a population of 3,000 divided into 1,500 households. One-person households may present special public health challenges, especially if the person is in the senior-citizen age group.

Because most people spend one- to two-thirds of their lives at home, housing has a profound influence on the health of the population, including the growth and development of children and the functioning of families. Households considered crowded or substandard in one community may be acceptable in another community. The amount of owner-occupied housing as opposed to renter-occupied housing often is used to indicate the stability and investment of residents in making their community a safe and attractive place to live. In some communities, however, renters are highly invested in their neighborhoods—both emotionally and economically—and are as vigilant as owners are in maintaining the quality of their buildings and their community.

THE SOCIAL ORGANIZATION OF A COMMUNITY

In Healthy People 2020, one of the overarching goals includes creating social and physical environments that promote good health for all groups. Social environments are linked to health related quality of life and life satisfaction. According to the U.S. Department of Health and Human Services in Healthy People 2010:

> The social environment has a profound effect on individual health, as well as on the health of the larger community, and is unique because of cultural customs; language; and personal, religious or spiritual beliefs. (p. 19)

The three lenses through which we will describe and analyze the social relationships and interactions that comprise the community's culture are as follows:

- Community institutions

- Horizontal stratification of the community

- Vertical segmentation of the community

COMMUNITY INSTITUTIONS

Institutions are standardized patterns of social behavior typified by a regular cycle of activities, specific groupings and personnel, and an accompanying set of rules and ideology. The presence and ongoing functioning of institutions give a community its character and its sense of permanence. When an activity or a social behavior is institutionalized, it is no longer dependent on a specific person or persons to make it happen. Rather, it has taken on a life of its own. The institution of marriage is a good example. It is not something each individual invents as he or she reaches adulthood. It is an established social pattern. And although each person has a choice of whether or not to partake in the institution of marriage, it is nonetheless clearly established as a normative expectation of adult life in our society. Marriage has a set of rules, both formal and informal, that govern its performance. Formal rules relate, for example, to who can marry, the age at which a person can become married without parental consent, and who can officiate at a marriage. Less formal rules, on the other hand, might govern the appropriate age difference between marriage partners or who may be invited to a wedding.

Because something is institutionalized does not mean it is incapable of change. It simply means change will require some kinds of societal reorganization. Using the same example, it is easy to see that the institution of marriage has undergone remarkable change within the past 30 years. These changes include the following:

- The age at which many people are choosing to marry

- The ease with which a divorce is obtained

- The roles each of the partners assumes

- The number of times people are married

Moreover, new institutions always are developing to meet societal needs that currently are not being addressed by existing institutions. The changing pattern of marriage in our society has created a need for standardized ways of dealing with divorce and the custody of children. Because divorce was less common in the past, the activities and rules surrounding becoming unmarried were not standardized, and each couple was left to work out a solution in their own way, on their own terms.

The community inquiry does not attempt to cover all aspects of culture, nor all the institutions that constitute a community's culture, but rather the major categories of institutions that one is likely to find in almost all communities. They also are the ones most useful for guiding public health practice. They include economic, government, domestic, religion, education, and recreational and voluntary institutions. Depending on the community, different institutions assume different levels of significance, and institutions not included in the list may be more important to your assessment. The critical factor is not a detailed account of every institution, but the ability to identify institutions and understand how they are linked to the health of the community. Health related institutions have been omitted, intentionally, from this section because they will be discussed in detail in Chapter 5, "Determining the Health of Your Community," which focuses exclusively on health, the health care infrastructure, and institutional health organizations.

Economic

Suggested Activity

Do the following:

- Describe the major economic base of the community—for example, manufacturing, industrial, wholesale, retail, resort, education, health, government center, commercial center, diversified.
- Describe the relationship between employers and employees or workers and management.
- List the major employers in the community.
- Describe the role of workers' association such as unions.
- Chronicle the changes in the economy over the last 10 years.
- Summarize the effect these economic changes have had on the community.
- Describe the health and safety factors associated with local industry.

Like all institutions, the economy of a community can be viewed both as cultural capital and as cultural liability. Economic leaders can be powerful allies in making communities healthy places in which to work, raise families, live in quality housing, receive an education, and grow old comfortably. At the same time, the health of a community may be endangered by an economy grounded in exploitation of specific populations, creating social and health disparities, or complicit in the degradation of the environment and natural resources. The degree to which economic opportunity, such as employment and financing, is available to all sectors of the population is an indication of the economic health of the community. Understanding the economy that fuels community life and the changes that have taken place over the years permits the most fundamental understanding of current and future health problems. These phenomena range from potentially dangerous ecological changes and environmental hazards to the physical, psychological, and social problems associated with low wages or unemployment (Worthman and Kohrt, 2005) or job loss (Burgard, Brand, and House, 2007; Grunberg, Moore, Sikora, and Greenberg, 2008; Sikora, Moore, Greenberg, and Grunberg, 2008). An assessment of health and safety factors of the local economy involves two components:

- Economic impact on the environment, including air, noise, water, and food pollution

- Economic influence on the health of citizens, including the conditions of employment, income, financial stress, and socioeconomic dislocations

In some communities, it is relatively easy to describe the local economy and its influence on community health, particularly if it has a single economic base—for example, a farming village, a tourist resort, or a manufacturing facility. In others, however, it may take several months or even years to reveal the true economic basis of a community. Many immigrant populations support their communities of origin with monthly remittances from relatives who have migrated to the United States. Similarly, communities may have an "underground" economy based on activities such as the sale of illicit drugs (Dreher, 1982b). In fact, the economic significance of such activities underlies much of the failure to reduce drug abuse in inner cities.

GOVERNMENT, POLITICS, AND LAW ENFORCEMENT

Suggested Activity

Do the following:

- Describe the formal structure of the local government.
- Identify local sources of public revenue (property tax, sales tax).
- Describe the election process.
- List the elected representatives for the community and their party affiliations.
- Summarize the political party representation in the community, including recent trends.
- Describe the law enforcement organization for the district.
- Describe the penal system.
- Summarize the government health department and officials responsible for overseeing the health of the community.
- Specify the local government's budget for health.
- Specify the voting records of elected officials on health issues.

Government is the official structure, set of activities, and officials entrusted with the authority to make decisions on behalf of the community and to create and enforce the laws and policies that administer the community. Politics is a system of social relations in which access to and exercise of power are played out, and where power is defined most elementally as the ability to influence. Although politics exists at every level of human organization, it is at the local level of government that people feel the effects most keenly. This is where governmental decisions enter the lives of citizens on a daily basis, such as the schools their children attend, the roads on which they drive, the police protection they receive, how their property is zoned, how waste is removed and sanitized, and the taxes they pay. A community culture inquiry must include the identity of local public officials, how they were invested with authority (elected, appointed, inherited), and how they vote on issues of health and welfare. This is essential information, both for explaining current health issues and for mobilizing the community for future health action. Political parties may or may not be represented at the most local level, and it is not uncommon to have two or three independent candidates running for office, each with his or her own agenda and constituency. On the other hand, many communities have a dominant political party affiliation that party leaders acknowledge through governmental assistance in return for community wide support.

The tax structure is the place in which economic institutions and political institutions come together. The concern of citizens over an increasing tax burden created by government initiatives—no matter how wholesome for the public they may be—is very real and can be a major deterrent in planning and implementing a healthy community agenda. The scattering of nuclear power plants throughout the northeast corridor of the United States in previous decades, for example, provided tax relief as well as employment opportunities for the citizens of small towns. Although this trend generated some local resistance—centered mainly on health and safety hazards for future generations—the short term tax reduction advantages to citizens were difficult to counter.

Domestic

Suggested Activity

Do the following:

- Describe the variation in domestic composition of households.
- Report the percentage of single-parent households.
- Determine the average number of children per household.
- Ascertain the expected roles of family members—for example, mother/father, husband/wife, child/parent, and child/grandparent.
- Describe the norms and rules governing courtship and marriage.
- Determine the legal age for marriage without parental consent.
- Find out the average age of first marriage.
- Report the rate of divorce, separation, and annulment.

The terms "household" and "family" often are used synonymously, generally because in American society, they often refer to the same group of people. For our purposes, however, family will refer to those related by kinship ties, whether by blood, adoption, marriage, or convention; and household will refer to those who share a living space. Although these are grossly oversimplified definitions, it is easy to see that depending on how family is defined, it is possible to have households composed of more than one family and families comprising more than one household. Communities differ greatly in the way their populations are organized into families and households. Some are divided into single household units, occupied by nuclear families consisting of a mother, a father, and their unmarried children. Others are much more complex and contain a variety of domestic arrangements. Extended families may occupy several households located in proximity, with extensive and routine visiting among them. In migrant-worker and refugee communities, it is not uncommon to have several unrelated individuals and families occupying the same household.

The household is just as important as the family. Households generally are composed of people who eat and sleep in the same dwelling and who are in routine (usually daily) contact. It is common for household members to have mutual caregiving functions, although it is not at all unusual for these functions to be shared by family members and others who are not part of the household. Because the household often is the unit of personal health care, trends in household structure and the implications for the health of the public are important to monitor.

The norms governing family, marital, and domestic life underpin some of our most ingrained institutions and often differ widely from culture to culture. It is imperative to set aside our own values regarding domestic life and not criticize how families are organized in households in other communities. For example, rather than supposing that the children of divorced parents are victims of a broken family, we could reframe them as children who have the benefit of belonging to two households with loving and protective parents. Moreover, in situations where there is only one parent, surrogate mothers and fathers often emerge from among friends, relatives, and neighbors to create a more healthful psychological environment than that which existed when the biological parents occupied the same household.

Another kind of family structure that has emerged over the past two decades is that of same-sex couples, including those who have publicly declared their commitment, share a residence, and sometimes raise children. Most recently, the right of same-sex couples to marry and/or form civil unions has been a significant issue, both socially and politically. Because the level of social acceptance of a gay/lesbian sexual orientation has been uneven, Healthy People 2010 set forth sexual identity and orientation as a topic in which health disparities occurred. In Healthy People 2020, lesbian, gay, transgender, and bisexual health has been added as a new topic area. For gay men, health issues include HIV/AIDS, substance abuse, depression, and suicide, while for lesbian women, some evidence points to higher rates of smoking, alcohol abuse, obesity, and stress. For both groups, personal safety and mental health are critically important issues (Healthy People 2020).

The social conventions pertaining to the sequence of courting, marriage, and pregnancy differ greatly from society to society. Marriage may be arranged without a period of courtship, and pregnancy may occur without marriage. In some cultures, it is common to attend a marriage ceremony in which all the children (and sometimes the grandchildren) of the couple are members of the wedding party. Traditions that may appear exotic to the outsider are supported in their communities (Dreher and Hudgins, 2010; McElroy and Townsend, 2004).

Religion

Suggested Activity

Do the following:

- List, by denomination, the churches, temples, and other places of worship attended by residents in the community and locate them on the map.

- Find out the size and average attendance of each congregation.

- Identify which churches are increasing in membership and which are decreasing.

- List the names of the clergy for the various churches.

■ Describe the role each religious facility plays in the health care of the community.

■ Identify the churches that have taken leadership positions for neighborhood or community health activity.

■ Identify any minority religious groups in the community.

The health of a community is heavily influenced by local religious institutions, both in the organization of services and as a vehicle of social and economic support for their members. Although many of the earlier direct care functions have disappeared, some religious groups or functionaries remain strong community advocates for health and bring considerable cultural capital to the public health table for senior-citizen–health promotion, care of preschool children, neighborhood improvement, and school violence abatement. The Catholic Church, for example, is the largest provider of non-government health care and education in the United States. Faith-based philanthropy such as Jewish Federation and Catholic Charities provide substantial community benefit to underserved populations and are important private-sector partners with local public health departments.

Many religious institutions play a significant role in reducing health disparities with funds, equipment, and health and social support services such as cooking and housekeeping, disease prevention, and health promotion activities. Even if they do not participate directly, religious institutions often lend their facilities to community health services such as after-school programs for teenagers, child day-care centers, senior centers, and sites for health fairs. Like other institutions, organized religions not only have buildings and activities, they also have leaders and officials who are likely to have considerable influence in the community and can support particular health projects. Religions are key institutions for resolving community health problems (Peterson, Atwood, and Yates, 2002).

Prevailing religious beliefs involving diet, pregnancy, family planning, and terminal illness must be considered in community health education and program development. Furthermore, certain religions may impose injunctions on common public health screening or prevention procedures. Finally, the relationship between religiosity and mortality, suggested 20 years earlier in the Alameda County Study by Berkman and Syme (1979), has been confirmed, with continued lower mortality rates for frequent attendees of religious services. This appears to be explained by improved health practices, increased social contact, and more stable marriages (Strawbridge, Cohen, Shema, and Kaplan, 1997), as well as more emotional support, a sense of spiritual connectedness, optimism, and better health in old age (Krause, 2002).

Education

Suggested Activity

Do the following:

- Describe the local governance of the public school system.
- Identify pre-college-level schools—both public and private—that serve the population and locate them on the map.
- Determine the approximate enrollment in each school or program.
- Describe the administration of the local public school system, including the following:
  - The function of the school board
  - The composition of the school board
  - How board members are elected or appointed
- Describe how the superintendent of schools is selected.
- List the names of the principal of each school.
- Describe the function and role of the school nurse.
- Describe other health services offered through the schools.
- Identify the educational institutions that are used for adult learning in the community.
- Identify the libraries and other educational facilities available to community residents.

The school system is an essential component of a community's cultural capital. In addition to traditional screening in the form of physical, vision, and hearing exams, health promotion is also carried out in schools, with educational programs for such issues as drug-abuse prevention, sex education, dental health, nutrition, and hygiene. School records on absenteeism provide an excellent source of data for case-finding and epidemiological investigations. Developing relationships with the principal and teachers of each school creates a foundation for efficiently reaching the majority of children in a community. Many states mandate the employment of a school nurse at both the elementary and secondary levels. The role of the school nurse encompasses the totality of the school health program, incorporating primary, secondary, and tertiary prevention strategies and creating a healthy school environment that provides a safe, supportive social environment and learning milieu for all children.

School boards differ in the degree of influence they exert on schools. Some retain great control of every aspect of school life, while others leave the administration to the principal and limit their input to financial matters. The composition and philosophy of the board will influence school health programs. In addition to getting to know the principal and teachers, it is important to meet the board members to enlist their support in building community capacity.

Adult education classes have become increasingly popular and provide an effective mechanism for offering health related courses such as emergency care, parenting, and stress reduction. Expert faculty members can assume a leadership role in promoting a healthy community agenda. The effectiveness of our schools and colleges and the ability of public health workers to reach all members of the community are central to public health.

Recreation

Suggested Activity

Do the following:

- Describe how community residents spend their leisure time.
- Locate and identify recreational areas and facilities. These include formal recreation facilities (for example, parks, playgrounds, theaters, zoos, golf courses, and public pools) and informal recreational facilities (for example, streets, vacant lots, and swimming holes).
- Locate publicly supported facilities, commercial facilities, and/or age-designated facilities (for example, for children, adolescents, senior citizens).
- Describe where children go to play.
- Post the parts of the day and week generally reserved for leisure activity.
- List the agencies and personnel specifically concerned with community recreation and leisure.

Play and recreation are important components of all societies. Recreation is directly related to health in its capacity for providing exercise, for meeting physical and psychological challenges, and as a form of relaxation and stress relief. The promotion of organized recreational activities, such as at supervised playgrounds and parks, has been a significant public health intervention for reducing accidents and promoting the safety of children. Recreation generates social interaction in the form of teams and clubs that can break down barriers and create the sense of unity that symbolizes a healthy community.

Recreation also includes books, magazines, radio, television, and the Internet. These recreational activities also serve a communication function and are important resources for public health education, particularly in the area of health promotion, prevention of disease, and personal management of health problems. The Internet provides ready access to a range of health information and rapid communication. Practically all women's and family magazines have health columns. Television shows, movies, soap operas, and novels deal with a variety of health problems, including driving while intoxicated, teenage suicide, drug abuse, family violence, living with chronic illness, Alzheimer's disease, and death and dying. Sensitively written and framed within the cultural experience of the audience, they can be a valuable teaching tool as well as a vehicle for mobilizing community action (for example, through a community reading program). The timing of health education or health screening programs to immediately follow a television drama that has generated the interest of the public can help to promote its success.

Although there are distinct advantages to recreational and leisure facilities for the purpose of promoting the health and safety of community residents, recreational institutions also generate community health problems. Recreational drinking, for example, can have serious consequences for communities. The safety and sanitation of public recreational facilities is another aspect of community practice. Broken bottles and rusty cans left in the park or on a beach can result in serious injuries. Some leisure and play activities place the participants at risk of personal injury and therefore require appropriate community resources to both prevent and manage potential injury. Although individuals and groups should not be prevented from the pleasures of mountain-climbing, scuba diving, running marathons, cycling, and football, they all carry considerable risk for injury and cost that may be borne by the community. Sports such as boating, snowmobiling, skiing, or skating may require public health initiated regulations, injury-prevention programs, and trauma services.

Voluntary

Suggested Activity

Do the following:

- Identify the voluntary organizations in the community by type:
  - Social
  - Economic
  - Religious
  - Educational
  - Political
  - Recreational
- Identify the leaders of each organization.
- Identify when, where, and how often they meet.
- Identify informal associations and groups within the community.

A culturally acceptable and efficient way to establish partnerships for action is to engage existing community groups. Voluntary associations are very important in building community capacity. They represent strength in both leadership and membership that can be readily deployed by community nurses to solve community problems and promote community health. Each of the institutions already discussed has its own voluntary associations consisting of groups of individuals who are bound together by a common interest. Therefore, there are many kinds of voluntary associations based on their stated purposes. One category, for example, consists of those based on common socio-demographic characteristic such as age (teen groups, young adults), ethnicity (Polish-American clubs, Sons of Cuba), and attendance at the same school (alumni associations, fraternities and sororities). Often, local branch associations are tied into national organizations and are highly formalized, such as the Masons or Elks clubs. Organizations that are national or international in scope are important resources for obtaining support from outside the community.

Typical economic voluntary associations are the Chamber of Commerce, trade associations, professional societies, or Kiwanis clubs. Occupational groups form to control and oversee various aspects of their trade or profession. Government and political associations, political-party branch organizations, and citizens' councils such as the League of Women Voters usually function to influence legislation locally and/or nationally. Voluntary associations also provide protective services such as fire and police protection. Parent-teacher associations are perhaps the best-known of all educational voluntary associations, but others include voluntary library service and bookmobiles, as well as travel societies, book clubs, and honor societies. Organized religion has led the way in establishing voluntary associations to carry on community activities. Church brotherhoods or women's committees, YMCA, YWCA, B'nai B'rith, and Jewish community centers are all examples of religious voluntary associations. Many recreational and artistic activities also are organized on a voluntary basis, including athletic clubs, choruses, bridge clubs, dance and theater groups, and chamber-music ensembles.

Voluntary groups ordinarily are formalized with titles and charters, regular meetings, and criteria for membership. There are other groups, however, that are more informally organized but equally important. These include teenagers who routinely meet in the local shopping mall, elders who eat breakfast at the same restaurant every morning, and men who gather each evening on a street corner or play chess in the park. Even though such informal groups are more difficult to identify and appear to be leaderless, they may have even more community influence than formal groups, and provide a constituency that could lend valuable support in creating and implementing a culturally informed healthy community agenda.

Practically all voluntary associations serve functions beyond their stated purpose, including lobbying politicians or helping members acquire jobs or borrow money. In addition, holding offices in voluntary organizations gives people a chance for leadership opportunities and status. Many join voluntary associations as a form of recreation, even if the goals of the association are not recreational. Voluntary associations also help newcomers to the community fit in and meet others with similar interests. Voluntary associations provide social guidance, imposing injunctions on the behavior of members and requiring that they conform to specific standards. Alcoholics Anonymous, for example, and other self-help groups have blossomed into a panorama of mutual assistance and support, gaining public support for addressing health problems such as obesity, smoking, cancer, muscular dystrophy, diabetes, and Alzheimer's disease. Many groups focused on health issues and problems were inspired and organized on the local level by nurses who recognized that individuals could relate therapeutically to others with the same problem and learn from them, knowing they had undergone a similar experience.

HORIZONTAL STRATIFICATION

Differences in wealth and status exist in practically all communities, no matter how small and homogeneous they first appear. These differences, when examined at the population level, constitute social classes of people that correlate more or less closely with income, educational level, and occupation. Social class represents categories of people of similar social rank having positions, responsibilities, possessions, and accomplishments of a more or less equal level and value.

Suggested Activity

Do the following:

- Describe the major socioeconomic levels in the community.
- Identify the socio-demographic variables and social institutions that distinguish the levels.

For those who are unfamiliar with a particular community, patterns of class stratification and socioeconomic differences between residents may be barely distinguishable, particularly if it is a community in which all citizens have limited access to resources. Often residents will actually deny the existence of social classes in their communities. Even so, the recognition of socioeconomic differences is of critical importance in understanding the community's social structure and power relationships. The differences that exist on the community level may not always—in fact, often do not—reflect the class differences that exist on the national level. They are nevertheless consequential for the community and are acknowledged by community members.

Most residents have an awareness of their position in relation to others. It is difficult to find a community where differences in status, income, and access to scarce resources do not exist. Even though classes are not formally organized groups, like voluntary associations, they have lives of their own. People enter them through birth or marriage or, with some difficulty, through the acquisition of socioeconomic resources and power as they progress through life. Although there is no formal membership process for entering a class, to be counted among a specific rank requires that others judge you to be so. This acceptance often is more difficult to obtain than the more formal membership of voluntary associations.

Generally, it is assumed that income, family name, occupation, residence, and education guide the social ranking of individuals. This is not always the case, however, as the criteria for determining social rank vary from community to community. Any member of the community may assume symbols of high social status such as manner of dress, etiquette, residence, and car, but these symbols do not mean the person is actually a member of that class. Moreover, the upper echelons, as well as members of their own social rank, may criticize such people for trying to imitate those of higher social rank. Nor can one assume that wealth and a profession will automatically qualify a resident for a particular social class. Although the actual ranking of individuals or households in terms of their socioeconomic status is not within the scope of this book, we can learn much about the culture of a community simply by the way people group themselves for social interaction—particularly in the areas of recreation and education. Because friendships and social activities often tend to follow class lines, the task of delineating socioeconomic strata for a particular community is not as difficult as one may anticipate. Although church memberships may embrace a wide range of social levels and the workplace may include all ranks present in the community, it is less likely that people of different classes will socialize routinely. The presence of private schools in a community along with the public school system also provides some clues as to how individuals rank themselves and each other. The horizontal stratification of the community will reveal the most fundamental power structure of the community. The support of people in the upper strata of the community is extremely helpful in accessing certain kinds of cultural capital and building-community capacity. The same people, however, also can be serious obstacles or threats to community health action.

VERTICAL SEGMENTATION

Suggested Activity

Do the following:
- Identify the vertical divisions of the community by type.
- Describe them in terms of differences in their institutions and socio-demographic characteristics.

In contrast to horizontal stratification, vertical segmentations are those sectors in the community that are not necessarily related to socioeconomic status or classes, but that nevertheless organize the community into subgroups. Depending on the community, these could be organized according to racial, ethnic, residential, religious, political, or occupational factors. A familiar example of vertical segmentation is the urban neighborhood composed of two or more dominant subgroups—such as Irish and Italian or African-American and Puerto Rican—each of which may express a full range of class or socioeconomic differentiation. Even though they may live side by side, the two groups may vote for different political candidates, have different social clubs, participate in different recreational activities, belong to different religions, and enjoy a different family life. Although they may intermingle on a daily basis, when there is a dispute between representatives of the two factions, it is likely they will support their respective ethnic groups.

Although those within these diverse segments share a common affiliation, they are rarely homogeneous, with social class, age, and religious differences prompting differences in values and lifestyles. Segment boundaries are permeated through marriage and childbearing so that some residents eventually claim membership in more than one social segment. These are important residents because they often have influence that spans the whole community. Such vertical segmentation is not limited to ethnic groups. Communities may be divided by characteristics such as residence (home renters versus owners), politics (Republicans, Democrats, and independents), or religion (Christians, Jews, and Muslims). Traditional conflicts between farmers and ranchers suggest similar factions based on occupation and a result of competition for land and water. In some cases, vertical segmentation is not easily discovered, and only becomes evident in times of conflict.

Similar to classes, vertical segments are not formally organized groups in the sense of having a regular charter, membership status, formal leadership, explicit rules of behavior, or routine meetings. Rather, they arise when a group of citizens has something in common that makes them different from another such group within the community. Despite the lack of officers, there often is a charismatic leader who is heartily endorsed by other members of the group, who is highly persuasive, has the ability to sway large numbers of people, and who controls citizen action, including elections.

For many people, the term "community" implies relationships of equality among its members. This discussion of social organization clearly shows that communities are in fact complex entities, made up not just of an environment and people but also of diverse institutions, classes, and groups with interests and goals that are sometimes shared and sometimes in conflict. It is important to know which segments of the community can be counted on to support a particular project and which cannot. It also is important to know which themes and activities unite community residents of various classes and segments and which separate them. It may be difficult, for example, to change public policy unless all the dominant segments of a multicultural community support the effort. The strategies for mobilizing citizen action for capacity building will be discussed in Chapter 6, "Laying the Foundation for a Healthy Community Agenda," and Chapter 7, "Leading Culturally Informed Community Action."

Unlike the tangible physical environment and unlike people, we cannot see or touch a class, an institution, or a vertical segment. A series of diagrams depicting the horizontal stratification and vertical segmentation in relation to each other and to community institutions can be very helpful to illustrate the social system and its points of intersection and cleavage. If, for example, the class structure were diagrammed according to religious institutions, it might be found that in some communities, all social levels attend the same church. This would thus be a point of intersection in the community—that is, a place where the nurse could reach a broad range of community residents as opposed to a specific segment.

Suggested Activity

Diagram the horizontal and vertical stratification of your community to look for points of intersection and points of separation, as in the following example.

HORIZONTAL STRATIFICATION IN A SMALL TOWN WITH A SINGLE-PURPOSE ECONOMY

Stratum	Religion	Economy	Schools	Recreation	Domestic	Housing
Upper elite	Catholic Anglican	Factory owner Professional Business	Private schools Catholic schools	Tennis Golf Sports fans Health clubs	Nuclear Older couples Single parent	Owners Large single family
Middle class	Methodist Catholic Baptist	Managers Commercial Teachers Government Trades	Public schools Catholic schools Private schools	Camping Sports fans Running	Nuclear Single parent	Owners Renters New tract housing
Working class	Catholic	Factory workers Unemployed	Public schools Catholic schools	Bowling league Sports fans	Large extended Single parent	Owners Renters

VERTICAL SEGMENTATION IN AN URBAN COMMUNITY UNDERGOING GENTRIFICATION

Institution	Indigenous Sicilian Families	Newcomers
Religion	Catholic	Various religions
Economy	Dock workers Local merchants Hospital workers Trades	Business people working out of neighborhood Artists
Education	High school Trade schools	Professional degrees College graduates
Recreation	Eastside bars	Westside clubs
Family	Large, extended, relatives nearby	Single person Couples and one-child families
Housing (city brownstones)	Owners	Renters/owners

Even though the community's health status has not been addressed directly, many potential problems and concerns can be identified simply by looking at its environment, its people, and the way in which they are organized and relate to their environment. This inquiry into the culture of a community not only exposes current health problems and predicts future ones, it also reveals the strengths and cultural capital that can be activated through citizen participation to build community capacity in the most culturally informed way.

DETERMINING THE HEALTH OF YOUR COMMUNITY

A healthy community is one that is grounded in a wholesome environment, promotes social justice and inclusiveness, and prevents and responds to health risks and problems in a timely and culturally informed manner. This chapter provides a systematic format for assessing the health of a community's environment, the population, and the effectiveness of the ideological and institutional health organizations available to address health concerns and create a healthy community.

CHAPTER 5 OBJECTIVES

- Learn to describe and analyze the health of a community.

- Apply a systematic and comprehensive procedure for assessing the health of a community.

- Compare the health of the community in different time periods and with other communities.

- Examine the community's health care infrastructure in terms of primary, secondary, and tertiary prevention.

- Examine the range of local beliefs and values related to health and healing.

COMMUNITY HEALTH ASSESSMENT

The community health assessment complements and completes the community culture inventory and documents not only the community's needs but also the resources that must be accessed to achieve the goals of Healthy People 2020. Communities are dynamic organizations in which both the strengths and the opportunities for improvement constantly change. Like the examination of community culture, community health assessment is an ongoing process of documenting, comparing, and analyzing environmental, population, and health organization indicators. Similar to the community culture inventory framework in Chapter 4, "Discovering the Culture of Your Community," the community health assessment in this chapter is organized according to environment, population, and social organization—specifically the organization of health and health care. The community health assessment schedule is not exhaustive. Depending on the community, components of the assessment will be more or less useful. Also, in some cases, additional kinds of information may be needed to understand and address community health issues, problems, and the resources available to address them. We encourage you to use the Healthy People 2020 website to supplement your review of community health statistics and resources as you do your health assessment.

ENVIRONMENTAL HEALTH

The culture inquiry in Chapter 4 identified topographical, meteorological, and climatic features of the environment that may place a community at risk for widespread health problems. Urbanization; the invention of the automobile, telephone, and computers; and the development of nuclear technology have drastically altered the temporal and spatial dimensions of cultures throughout the world. The rapid changes over the past two centuries have intensified global warming and pollution, and necessitated public health action.

Ensuring the health of a community requires ensuring the health of the environment. In the aftermath of an earthquake and the subsequent cholera outbreak in Haiti in 2010, departures from environmental standards for cleanliness and safety precipitated serious health problems and compromised the most essential requirements to sustain life—air, water, and food—as the disaster affected dwellings, the workplace, communication, and transportation. Improving the quality of the environment improves the health of residents and the relationships among them. Healthy People 2020 includes environmental health as one of its major topic areas with the following six themes:

- Outdoor air quality

- Surface- and ground-water quality

- Toxic substances and hazardous waste

- Homes and communities

- Infrastructure and surveillance

- Global environmental health

The influence of the environment on health is not a new topic in public health (Armelagos, Brown, & Turner, 2005). Natural forces such as volcanoes, dust storms, weather depressions, floods, and insect pests have altered air, water, and food supplies in ways that have threatened human life. Over the centuries, humans have burned wood and charcoal, causing localized air pollution. In 2007, for the first time, more than 50% of the global population lived in urban areas (WHO, 2007). It is the process of urbanization that has most likely placed the environment at greatest risk. Pollution and cities go hand in hand as large congregations of people strain the environment. Overcrowding and environmental overload exhaust environmental resources, and high-density populations often are associated with industrial activity that adulterates soil, water, and air with various forms of solid and gaseous contaminants. Foul odors, dirty streets and roads, unkempt housing, and unclean recreational areas all give the impression of people that have lost interest in the place where they live, work, and play. The effect is dismal and promotes a negativism that pervades the community. On the other hand, a beautiful environment that is uncluttered and pleasing to the senses is not only a signal, but also a source of community health.

Safeguarding the environment for the health of the public is an international problem. Even remote contamination sites affect communities located thousands of miles away. In 2011, when the nuclear facilities in Japan were damaged as a result of an earthquake and the ensuing tsunami, all the local residents were removed from the area around the power plants, and citizens on the west coast of the United States also took precautions against contamination. Effective environmental health in even a small community in northern Japan may generate health risks in national and global arenas. International collaboration must be initiated to lower the levels of carbon dioxide emissions, manage the production and storage of nuclear waste, limit worldwide population growth to sustainable levels, and address the economic inequities that plague the world environment. These four factors are implicated in the self-perpetuating cycle of ecological degradation found worldwide (Friedman, 2008).

The assessment of the environment in the following pages is, again, by no means exhaustive. Rather, it is simply a guide to some of the most common environmental health problems. The relevance and prioritization of problems will vary from community to community. Industrialized societies, for example, will be concerned with nuclear contamination, while agricultural communities may be more concerned with soil contamination, pesticide runoff, insect control, and potable water.

Outdoor Air Quality

Suggested Activity

Do the following:

- Record the air-quality index in the community.
- Describe the measures being put into place to reduce the risk of adverse health effects caused by air pollution.
- Identify the actual and potential sources of air pollution.
- List the major modes of transportation in the community.
- Identify the topographical or climatic features that interact with sources of air pollution and augment the problem.

■ List local health problems that are attributable to air pollution.
■ Show the trends over the past 20 years regarding air pollution.
■ Compare these trends to state, national, and international levels.
■ Identify the populations disproportionately affected by air pollution.

The quality of the air is a major factor in promoting the health and survival of the human community. Exposure to air pollution contributes to a variety of health problems such as asthma, emphysema, lung cancer, and other chronic lung diseases. Although most health problems associated with air pollution affect the respiratory system, eye irritation and dermatological reactions also are common.

Air pollution is a result of contamination of the atmosphere by airborne substances that are potentially harmful to humans as well as to animals and plants. For centuries, people have burned wood and its derivatives for cooking and for heat, thus emitting ash, smoke, soot, and dust into the air. It was during the industrial revolution in England, however, that contamination of the air received the greatest attention from public health officials, inspiring movements to regulate the burning of coal to control the amount of smoke and soot. Polluting particulate matter has expanded from the derivatives of wood to include aerosol droplets, pesticides, insecticides, and herbicides. Cigarette-smoking, traditionally considered a personal health problem, has now assumed significance as a public health problem, as research has confirmed that the noxious components of tobacco smoke are damaging not only to those who smoke, but also to those who are exposed to tobacco-smoking by others.

Approximately 58% of the population in the United States lives in communities where outdoor air-pollution levels are dangerous to health, with the poor at higher risk (American Lung Association, 2010). The respiratory consequences of air pollution are mediated by the weather. Acid aerosols are worse in the winter in areas where coal-fired industry is common. Oxidates, including atmospheric ozone, are worse in the summer, especially midday to late afternoon when the sun is the hottest. Some of the illnesses related to air pollution include bronchitis, pneumonia, and the acute exacerbation of cardiopulmonary disease, asthma, and chronic obstructive pulmonary disease (COPD).

Today, the major sources of air pollution are emissions from motor vehicles, industry, and energy production. The emission of noxious gases such as carbon monoxide, carbon dioxide, and sulfur dioxide from petroleum and coal combustion and chlorofluorocarbons (CFCs) from propellant spray cans, solvents, and refrigerants has contributed to contamination of the air. These gases are hypothesized to contribute to an intensified greenhouse effect by depleting ozone in the stratosphere, which provides a vital protective layer against lethal irradiation. If the predicted global warming resulting from the increase in greenhouse gases actually takes place, the consequences for health and human survival could be catastrophic (Friedman, 2008; McMichael, 2001).

Although controversy about the timing, cause, and extent of global warming continues, there is little debate about its effect on rainfall, ground water, food production, and ozone depletion. Topographical factors and climatic conditions interact with sources of air pollution to create even more pernicious and widespread problems. Mexico City, Denver, and Los Angeles, for example, have particularly serious problems because of topographical features that trap polluted air over the most populated areas. Communities that lie in a river valley often are subject to air inversion—that is, the trapping of warm air on the ground by cooler air higher up, a common occurrence in valley ecologies. It is not unusual for the level of air pollution in such communities to be incompatible with national standards.

Surface- and Ground-Water Quality

Suggested Activity

Do the following:

- Identify the proportion of persons in the community who meet the standards set in the Safe Drinking Water Act.
- Identify the source of the public water supply.
- Find out the proportion of households using private water supplies.
- Describe the process that is used to treat the water supply.
- Report the frequency of water supplies inspected.

- Identify unsatisfactory water reports over the past five years.
- Locate on a map and date episodes of outbreaks of disease due to water pollution over the past five years.
- Report industrial or human waste being discharged into local water.
- Describe fluoridation policies.
- Identify the populations disproportionately affected by water pollution.

A safe and adequate water supply is essential to the health and survival of a population. From early times, water has been a vehicle for the disposal of waste. Communities may pollute rivers, streams, and lakes with sewage disposal and industrial byproducts, contaminating the water sources of communities downstream. In most industrialized societies, the bacteriologic infections carried by water, such as cholera, have been greatly reduced or eliminated through water-treatment processes, including the addition of chlorides. The pollution of both surface and ground water by industrial waste, however—including radioactive materials and lethal chemical byproducts—is cause for concern.

An environmental assessment to ensure the potability—or drinkability—of water includes both the public water supply and private springs or wells. Affecting every continent, water scarcity and inadequate sanitation are an increasing global concern (United Nations, 2010). Lack of sanitation causes diseases such as cholera, dysentery, and other diarrheal problems, a leading cause of childhood mortality. Clean water supplies also are important for recreation, such as swimming and boating, and commerce, such as fishing. The addition of chemicals to the public water supply has been a much-debated public health issue, particularly with reference to fluorides. On the other hand, the increase in dental-health problems due to unfluoridated water supply also is a public health problem. A Healthy People 2020 recommendation is to increase the percentage of persons served by community water systems, identifying households not using the public water supply as at-risk for dental-health problems. Herbicides and pesticides used in agriculture also are potentially harmful pollutants, and water in such communities, as well as those bordering and downstream, require testing specifically for these products.

Food Contamination

Suggested Activity

Do the following:

- Locate and date outbreaks or episodes of illness as a result of unsanitary or adulterated food products.
- Identify pesticides and herbicides used to protect local food crops.
- Identify food-garden sites near contaminated water, soil, or air.
- Identify populations disproportionately affected by food contamination.

The contamination of food can be caused by a variety of pollutants in the air, water, or soil. Dumping dangerous chemical waste products pollutes water and contaminates local fish products. The use of pesticides and herbicides is a threat to those who handle them, and downstream water supplies are often toxic. DDT, one of the most commonly used pesticides, is so toxic it was banned in the early 1970s. Public health concerns over outbreaks of infection from food and milk contamination have now shifted to problems created by the adulteration of food products. In addition to chemical fertilizers, the purposeful addition of other nonfood ingredients to enhance the flavor, augment the color, increase the size, and improve the shelf life of a product all are examples of food adulteration, the impact of which on health is only partially known.

TOXIC SUBSTANCES AND HAZARDOUS WASTE MANAGEMENT

The ability to create a safe and healthful environment for a flourishing community requires the management of various forms of contaminants and other hazardous wastes, such as sewage, solid waste, lead, chemical and pesticide byproducts, and radioactive materials. Uncontrolled dumping of waste poses a serious threat to the air, water, and food necessary to support human life and the aesthetics to enhance it.

Solid Waste

Suggested Activity

Do the following:

- Identify sources of solid wastes.
- Describe where and how solid wastes are disposed and/or recycled.
- Record community health problems within the past five years as a result of solid wastes.
- Describe compliance of solid-waste disposal with federal, state, and local regulations.
- Map and date public recreational facilities (parks, campgrounds, or beaches) condemned within the last five years as a result of solid-waste dumping.
- Map breaches of sanitary codes in the last five years.
- Map areas where disposal of trash and garbage is a visible problem.

The dark side of postwar technology resulting in disposable and non-biodegradable materials can be found in the litter of bottles, cans, and plastic containers that pollute the land and seascapes. The collection and disposal of solid wastes and unwanted byproducts of industry are major public health problems, not only because of the potential contamination of water and food supplies, but also because of the risk to animals and the unsightliness of the environment. Odoriferous and rat-infested dumps create both a health and an aesthetic problem for community residents. As landfills reach capacity, financial and political controversies have emerged. It is not unusual for residents to oppose new plans for solid-waste–disposal sites. Illegal dumping has become a criminal activity, but often is outside the control of local public health authorities.

Sewage

Suggested Activity

Do the following:

- Describe local methods for eliminating sewage.
- Identify local cultural practices and beliefs related to the elimination of fecal waste.
- Identify sources of sewage contamination in the environment.
- Describe sewage-management compliance with local, state, and federal codes.
- Map and date outbreaks of disease or other health problems attributed to problems in the management of sewage during the last five years.
- Identify populations disproportionately affected by sewage contamination.

Every culture and community has firmly established patterns for the disposal of human wastes and the management of fecal materials. As with other forms of pollution, urbanization has limited the facilities available for adequate sewage disposal in densely populated settlements. Rural communities also require vigilance regarding the management of human waste. Septic tanks leach fields, and cesspools are used in rural areas and inspected regularly. As with other forms of waste, the management of sewage has both health and aesthetic implications. Water-borne diseases such as giardia, cholera, and amoebiasis are the direct result of contamination by fecal material, either animal or human.

Radioactive Waste

Suggested Activity

Do the following:

- Map documented radioactive contamination in the community.
- Describe the role of community in transport, storage, and/or disposal of radioactive materials.
- Describe the level of compliance in management of radioactive materials with federal and state regulations.
- Map public health problems attributable to nuclear/radioactive exposure within the last five years.
- Compare rates of cancer, particularly leukemia, to state and national rates.
- Describe social or psychological problems associated with nuclear exposure.
- Identify populations disproportionately exposed to radiation.

Although there are millions of contaminants that, in certain quantities, can be damaging to the health of a population, radioactive substances probably have received the most attention in recent years, particularly as the need for energy increases. Everyone is exposed to some form of radiation simply through natural contact with the cosmic rays of the sun and substances of the earth. More dangerous levels of exposure come from medical X-rays, uranium mining and processing, nuclear-power plants, and nuclear-weapons development. The production, transportation, storage, and disposal of radioactive materials, such as nuclear fuel, present a significant health and safety hazard. Furthermore, the contamination of groundwater supplies can spread the danger far beyond the local community. Since the development of the nuclear-weapons industry at the end of World War II, radioactive materials have been released into our environment.

The disposal of nuclear waste, given the long half-life of many of its toxic products, is a foremost public health concern. Various states have raised objections in Congress to the mass transfer of nuclear waste to be stored within their borders.

As with other forms of waste, cases of illegal dumping of nuclear material place the public at risk in spite of government regulation. The potential for sabotage and accidents in the storage and transport of nuclear materials poses both physical and psychological threats. There are many health risks associated with exposure to radiation, including leukemia and other forms of cancer, genetic mutations, and fetal damage. Careful records reporting the incidence of such diseases and health problems from year to year provide important data regarding potential radioactive contamination.

Chemical and Pesticides

Suggested Activity

Do the following:

- Map sources of chemicals and pesticides in the community.
- Identify the percentage of children with elevated blood-lead levels.
- Determine how many provider visits are attributable to chemical and pesticide exposure.
- Describe compliance of chemical and pesticide management with federal and state guidelines.
- Identify evidence of uncontrolled or illegal dumping.
- Identify health problems or outbreaks of disease attributed to chemicals and pesticides in the last five years.
- Identify social or psychological problems attributed to exposure to chemicals and pesticides.
- Map nearby Superfund sites.
- Identify populations that are disproportionately exposed to chemicals and pesticides.

Although not a new problem, the pollution of the environment from dangerous chemical waste first received serious public attention with the Love Canal incident in the early 1970s (Levine, 1982). Hazardous chemicals were leaching from an abandoned disposal site located in an old canal where an elementary school had been built. Because the disposal had begun in the 1940s and was decades old, most residents of this newly thriving community in upstate New York were unaware of the disposal site's proximity to the area where their homes were built. After moving into their homes, the chemical pollution traveled through underground waterways into yards and basements, and vaporized into the air. After extensive media attention and political involvement, studies were conducted that revealed an excessive miscarriage rate, although other health risks were not so definitively implicated. Many people moved their families from this site, and many more became aware of the difficulty of addressing suspected environmental problems (Newton and Smith, 2004).

Similar problems were encountered with Agent Orange, a defoliant used in the Vietnam War. Exposure to chemical-warfare agents in Iraq during Desert Storm was suspected of causing health problems, which the press dubbed "Gulf War Syndrome." The uncontrolled dumping of chemical wastes through the past century and the illegal dumping of more recent years continue to pose major health problems for the nation. The National Priorities List, also known as the Superfund sites, scores hazardous-waste sites by a hazard-ranking system. There are more than 1,400 Superfund sites in the United States, and the Agency for Toxic Substances and Disease Registry (ATSDR) assesses their potential for health effects. This federal program, designed to clean up huge sites of chemical, nuclear, and industrial waste, was established by Congress in 1980. Superfund sites are designated by the Environmental Protection Agency (EPA).

Each day, new research findings suggest exposure to dangerous chemicals and pesticides is the etiology of many health problems, including various forms of cancer, birth defects, neurological disorders, reproductive problems, immunological disturbances, gastrointestinal problems, dermatological diseases, and vision problems (Healthy People 2020). For example, human exposure to lead can cause problems such as hypertension, anemia, kidney damage, learning disabilities, and impaired fetal development. Increased levels of lead in the environment occur by corrosion of leaded water pipes as well as from manmade products such as car batteries, cables, pipelines, lead-based paints, pesticides, ceramic glazes, candles, cigarette smoke, and the glass in computer and television screens. Although we know about the hazardous effects of lead, only roughly 20% of the approximately 60,000 industrial chemicals used in this country have been tested for their toxic potential to human health. Sources of exposure include water contamination, lawn fertilizers, contaminated food and dairy products, pesticides and herbicides, and some disinfectants. In a study of 270 pregnant women, detectable levels of 163 chemicals were found in 100% of the women, and perchlorate (a regulated chemical used in propellants for rockets and explosives) was found in 99% to 100% of the women (Woodruff, Zota, and Schwartz, 2011). The exposure of pregnant and lactating women, infants, and young children to these products is thought to be correlated with birth defects and blood dyscrasias, including leukemia. Healthy People 2020 recommends monitoring blood and urine to measure the recommended reduced exposure to chemicals such as arsenic, cadmium, lead, mercury, chlordane, DDT, and others. It is critically important not only to monitor the effects of hazardous chemicals, but also to advocate for their removal.

Noise Pollution

Suggested Activity

Do the following:

- Map areas of noise pollution.
- Describe health problems attributable to noise pollution.
- Describe enforcement of regulations related to the control of noise.
- Identify populations disproportionately exposed to noise pollution.

An often-overlooked public health problem is noise. Noise pollution is a byproduct of our advanced industrialization and technology. Although research in the area of noise pollution is comparatively new, it is now known to contribute not only to hearing loss, but also to stress reactions, irritability, cardiac disease, high blood pressure, and accidents. The public must be educated regarding the potential damage of self-inflicted exposure to noise, such as power boating or loud music, and formulate and implement policies to control the amount of public noise created by aircraft, motor vehicles, and other noise pollutants.

Disease Vectors

Suggested Activity

Do the following:

- Map potential at-risk areas for vector-carried disease in the community.
- Map outbreaks of reportable vector-carried diseases.
- Map areas with rat infestation.
- List and date outbreaks of disease as a result of rat infestation.
- Map insect infestation.
- Describe community health risks associated with the following:
  - Mosquitoes
  - Houseflies
  - Cockroaches
  - Lice
  - Fleas
  - Ticks
  - Bedbugs
  - Biting flies
- Compare community trends in vector infestation with state and national trends.
- Identify populations disproportionately affected by disease-carrying vectors.

Although the emphasis in environmental health has shifted from food contamination and disease vectors to chemical, nuclear, and solid-waste pollution, the control of insects and rodents continues to be a public health problem in many communities, both in the United States and internationally. It is well-known that many diseases are transmitted to human populations by rats and/or various kinds of insects. The role of the mosquito in spreading malaria, yellow fever, dengue fever, West Nile virus, and other infectious diseases is the major incentive for massive mosquito-control programs in swampland areas. Cockroaches and houseflies are common offenders in transmitting gastrointestinal disease through the contamination of food. Insect vectors (agents) transmit disease by sucking the blood of the infected person or animal (host) and transmitting it to another person through deposits in food or through biting.

The vehicle for control of vector-transmitted disease is entering the sequence of infection at some point to break the chain of infection among host, agent, and environment. This includes several methods, such as destroying the breeding grounds of insects (drainage of swampland and household sanitation); exterminating rats that harbor disease-carrying fleas; and using insecticides and physical barriers such as repellents, nets, or screens. The selection of method depends upon the life cycle and natural habitat of both the agent and the host. Intervention must occur at both the community and household levels, including health education and inspection programs. In recent years, Lyme disease and other tick-borne illnesses have received increased attention.

Preparedness

Suggested Activity

Do the following:

- Obtain the local and state disaster plan for the community.
- Map and date potential disasters for the community.
- Identify the cultural capital relative to disaster response in the community.
- Describe the disaster responses to recent emergencies, identifying the following:
    - Local, state, and national involvement
    - Success of the disaster plan in preventing problems
    - Areas for improvement in local and state response capacity

The Federal Emergency Management Agency (FEMA), housed within the Department of Homeland Security, was established in 1979 to respond to emergencies that overwhelm local and state resources. As noted in Chapter 4, some communities are more at risk for disasters than others, and flooding, hurricanes, tornadoes, and earthquakes can be predicted, expected, monitored, and prepared for in an organized fashion. However, not all natural disasters are predictable; a level of community preparedness to anticipate such disasters is necessary to significantly reduce the consequences. According to Healthy People 2020:

> Preparedness involves Government agencies, nongovernmental organizations, the private sector, communities, and individuals working together to improve the Nation's ability to prevent, prepare for, respond to, and recover from a major health incident.

An increased emphasis on disaster preparedness has emerged recently as a response to the earthquakes and tsunamis in Southeast Asia and Japan, the hurricane in Louisiana, and the earthquake in Pakistan.

Although not natural disasters, the Oklahoma City bombing in 1995, the World Trade Center terrorist attacks in 1992 and 2001, and the anthrax contamination in 2001 alerted the nation to a kind of vulnerability previously unimagined. These human-produced disasters are less predictable, and preventing and preparing for them is less straightforward. FEMA, for example, designed a national plan to immunize all health care professionals against smallpox after 9/11 and the anthrax threat. One component of this plan was to recruit community health nurses as volunteers to National Disaster Medical System (NDMS) nurse response teams (NNRT) to implement a vaccination program. The plan, however, was never realized after various sectors questioned its wisdom and many individuals did not seek the vaccination.

All disasters have the potential to contaminate air and water; disseminate toxic bacteria in various ways; cause massive injury, death, and destruction; and induce pervasive fear, anger, and grief throughout communities. Therefore, local, state, national, and international disaster response plans are critical to safeguarding the environment, protecting the population's health, and instilling a sense of control and well-being in the face of overwhelming threat.

Crime

Suggested Activity

Do the following:

- List the 10 leading crimes in the community.
- Describe changes that have occurred in the kinds and frequency of crimes over the last 10 years.
- Map high-crime areas.
- Describe the incidence of reported crimes against children.
- Describe the incidence of reported crimes against older persons.
- Identify populations disproportionately affected by crime.

The safety of housing, workplaces, schools, streets, recreational areas, commercial centers, and other public areas requires vigilance and management to promote and protect the health of the public and create a context in which people feel secure. Personal injury crimes constitute a growing problem that has physical and psychological implications for the health of the public. Perhaps no other issue so dramatically illustrates the significance of the human environment in the health and well-being of populations. Poverty, unemployment, the availability of firearms, drugs, violence, victimization, racism, and sexism all have been correlated with the occurrence of personal injury crimes (Office of National Drug Control Policy, 2006) as well as a more-generalized fear of crime that inhibits healthy community interaction. The incidence of violent crimes against individuals, including murder, rape, robbery, and assault, varies among communities and populations. For some problems, such as domestic violence and incest, accurate statistics at the local level are very difficult to determine, and national statistics provide only estimations at the local level. Murder rates, on the other hand, are comparatively accurate. In the 1990s, firearm homicide was the leading cause of death for teenage African-American males (DuRant, Cadenhead, Pendergrast, Slavens, & Linder, 1994). Some 12 years later, young African-American males (age 15 to 24) had a rate of homicide three times that of young Hispanic men and 17 times that of young white men (Kaiser Family Foundation, 2006).

In addition to reducing related morbidity and mortality, Healthy People 2020 aims for a 10% reduction in firearm-related deaths. Public health efforts in relation to environments conducive to crime include identifying the risk factors and high-risk groups that are correlated with high crime rates. They also include the identification of high-risk behaviors, such as aggression in elementary and junior high–school students, and interventions to teach and model alternative means of conflict resolution.

In addition to having immediate and equal access to qualified protective services, all citizens of a community should have educational programs to help them avoid and report crimes and to rehabilitate victims of crime. The increase in the prison population in the United States reflects both an increase in crimes and the failure of jural-penal institutions, such as law enforcement and the courts, to respond effectively to this crisis. In addition to an aging inmate population, studies have found as many as 80% of prison inmates have substance-abuse problems, yet many penal systems do not have rehabilitation programs in place. The proportion of the prison population that is HIV-positive or has AIDS and tuberculosis is much higher than in the general population (Hammett, Harmon, and Rhodes, 2002). The problem of crime and society's response to it is controversial, including, for example, gun control. Public health has a pivotal role to play in prisons and schools as well as the responsibility to inform politicians who establish policy related to crime, personal safety, and the penal system.

Accidents

Suggested Activity

Do the following:

- List the type, number, and rate of accidents occurring in the community.
- Compare these figures with state and national levels.
- Describe trends over the past 10 years.
- Identify populations affected by each type of accident.

Accidents continue to be a leading cause of death in the nation, especially among young children, teenagers, and older adults. Motor-vehicle accidents are the most common cause of childhood injury. Alcohol use is highly correlated with motor-vehicle accidents, and this knowledge has inspired the now-common driver-education programs in high schools, safe-driver programs for more experienced motorists, laws governing the number of drinks and acceptable blood-alcohol levels, and the formation of the organization Mothers Against Drunk Driving (MADD).

The rate of falls resulting in hip fracture in those over 65 also constitutes a major public health problem, affecting women twice as much as men. Efforts to ensure prompt attention to accident victims, such as volunteer first-aid training, an emergency medical technician program, and adequate emergency transport, minimize the damage as much as possible and the untoward effects such as fear of falling, sedentary behavior, impaired function, and lower quality of life (Healthy People 2020).

The formulation of public policy and governmental regulation to prevent accidents is equally as important. Proper labeling and packaging of poisonous substances, seat-belt laws, and building regulations requiring window guards for young children are all examples of primary prevention policy. Making streets and highways safer for motorists and pedestrians; enforcing domestic and occupational safety codes to avoid accidents at home or in the workplace; and creating safe, protected recreational environments are essential to promote the health of a population.

Homes and Communities

Suggested Activity

Do the following:

- Describe the range of housing in the community.
- Describe compliance of housing with state and local regulations for safety, sanitation, and state of repair.
- Identify health risks presented by the condition of local housing.

- Map problems (accidents, fires, and outbreaks of diseases) attributed to poor housing.
- Identify populations disproportionately affected by substandard

In Chapter 4, the quantity, placement, and construction of housing in the community was addressed. In the community health assessment, indoor air pollution, adequate heating and sanitation, housing structure, and safety issues such as exposure to lead-based paint and electrical and fire hazards are the major concerns (Healthy People 2020). Because people spend a major portion of their lives in households, the type and condition of housing—including living space, cooking facilities, and privacy—have a profound impact on the health of the population, including the growth and development of children and family interaction. Poor or inappropriately constructed housing may contribute to disease, crime, or safety problems such as high rates of fires, falls, and other accidents.

Improving the health of a community is highly dependent on the quality of the domiciles in which residents live. Residents must be alerted to the potential hazards of existing housing. Advocacy at the policy level must be accomplished to raise the standard of housing in the community. The kinds of problems encountered in community health practice include lead paint in older housing, radon gas, neglected housing repairs, and safety hazards in the homes of elders as well as young families.

Community Buildings

Suggested Activity

Do the following:

- Describe compliance with local housing regulations.
- Describe enforcement of occupancy and activities regulation.
- Describe enforcement of nonsmoking rules.

- Describe compliance with OSHA standards for occupational safety and health.
- List accidents or outbreaks of disease attributable to breaches of health and safety standards in the workplace or other public buildings.
- Map buildings with health and safety problems.

Similar to the private space of the home, the public space of the school, workplace, and other community buildings must have a clean, safe, and acoustically and aesthetically pleasing inner environment. Most communities have codes regulating the capacity of buildings in terms of the number of people who can be there at any one time; the activities that can or cannot take place; the kind and quality of construction or renovation; and the health and safety factors of furnishings and installations such as plumbing, insulation, carpeting, paint, and wall covering. These regulations on the interior environment are for the protection of the public; breaches of the code require appropriate action. Code violations might include hoarding, poor lighting, sanitation violations in restrooms, nonenforcement of smoking regulations, improper ventilation, and inadequate climate control.

The workplace is one of the most significant public interiors. The majority of the adult workforce spends at least eight hours a day, five days a week, on the job, where they may be exposed to a variety of health hazards ranging from noise to dangerous chemicals to machinery. Similar to protecting and monitoring the natural environment, solving the problems of the workplace environment is complicated by the economic pressures facing many smaller industries as well as their employees. Even when workers are at risk for serious health problems as a result of some workplace feature, they may be reluctant to take unified action if they believe their livelihood will be threatened. Although the protection of workers' health is ultimately in the best interest of the company, employers may be reluctant or even unable to expend the necessary resources. Establishment of the Occupational Safety and Health Administration (OSHA), an agency in the Department of Labor, was intended to protect workers in such situations.

Energy Management

Suggested Activity

Do the following:

- List sources of energy, such as electricity, gas, oil, wood, and kerosene, used in the community.
- Identify major public sources of energy.
- Identify private sources of energy in the community.
- Describe the adequacy of public power sources.
- Identify wasted energy.
- List health/safety problems derived from major energy sources.

Urbanization, industrialization, and advanced technology require large amounts of energy to create an environment appropriate to the welfare and development of human populations. The conservation of energy is a public health problem that requires community wide education and governmental regulation. In addition to the dangers of nuclear energy already cited, power dams pose the threat of floods, and electricity poses the threat of electrocution and electrical fires. The increasing use of wood stoves and kerosene heaters to reduce costly fuel bills also poses the threat of pollution and fire. Both domestic and public management of fuel and energy resources require an educated public and enforcement of safety regulations when using these resources.

Global Health

Suggested Activity

Do the following:

- Identify professionals trained in global health and the detection/ management of global disease in the community.
- Identify the nearest CDC Global Disease Detection Regional Center.
- Describe human migration patterns in the community.

■ Find out the rate of tuberculosis for foreign-born persons.
■ Describe the range of perceptions regarding international persons/
groups in the community.

We live locally, but we are citizens of a larger planet, earth. Globalization—that
is, the unification of the people who make up our planet through migration and
communication—is not a new phenomenon, but it is occurring at a staggering
speed. Through technological advances in transportation and communication, we
can travel great distances in an increasingly shortened timeframe and communicate instantly almost anywhere in the world. Similarly, environmental health
issues and infections know no national boundaries. Global health is defined as
follows:

> ... an area for study, research, and practice that places a priority
> on improving health and achieving equity in health for all people
> worldwide. Global health emphasizes transnational health issues,
> determinants, and solutions; involves many disciplines within and
> beyond the health sciences and promotes interdisciplinary collabo-
> ration; and is a synthesis of population-based prevention with
> individual-level clinical care. (Koplan, Bond, Merson, Reddy,
> Rodriguez, et al., 2008, p. 1995)

Historically, migration patterns and colonization spread infectious disease, causing much loss of life such as with the Athenian plague (430 BCE), the Black
Death (1347 CE), and measles and smallpox epidemics among Native Americans
(17th century). Whether with respect to H1N1, cholera, or severe acute respiratory syndrome (SARS), an awareness of how we affect one another globally was
considered sufficiently important for the health of U.S. citizens that it was included as a new topic in Healthy People 2020. Furthermore, global health is important because of the unmeasured impact the United States has on the health of
other countries where the United States disposes wastes, such as batteries, computers, and other toxic items and substances. As global citizens, we have a
responsibility to know about global health issues and to advocate for a just and

good society—one that works to reduce the burden of disease related to poor water quality, sanitation, insufficient hygiene, dangerous policies, and inequitable access to global resources.

ENVIRONMENTAL HEALTH HIGHLIGHTS

This section highlighted of some of the major environmental resources, issues, and problems faced by communities in rural, urban, and global environments. The extent to which the environment can be protected from the pollution and contamination that accompany global urbanization is directly related to the sustainability of communities and the success future populations will achieve in obtaining optimum health and welfare. It is clear that for decades, very little thought was given to sustainability of the environment, and society is now paying the price. In a more optimistic vein, while advanced technology has contributed to the problem of environmental pollution, it is equally likely to reduce or eliminate pollution.

Legislation, policy, and economic sanctions are the major tools health workers use to promote healthy environments and to combat environmental problems. Thus, emission standards for motor vehicles, regulations on dumping chemical wastes, and bottle-recycling laws will have a greater impact on improving the quality of the environment and reducing the presence of disease, disability, and injuries than any one-to-one patient-care intervention. Many environmental problems require even broader-scale, multi-community action at the state, national, and global level. The movement of air and water, for example, carries contaminants across and through many communities, often far away from the origin of contamination and without reference to political boundaries. Effective control seldom can be sufficiently achieved by a local community. For this reason, the federal government has taken a major role in this dimension of public health. The EPA was established in 1970 to coordinate all activities that concern the quality of the environment—the atmosphere, land, and water. It has authority over the states and is responsible for conducting research, providing information, establishing and enforcing standards, and monitoring the quality of the environment.

OSHA was established to develop standards and coordinate safety and health oversight in the workplace. This federal agency regulates policy with regard to tuberculosis control in hospitals and is particularly important for nurses, who are one of the groups most affected by occupationally induced illness. The National Institute for Occupational Safety and Health (NIOSH), housed at the Centers for Disease Control and Prevention (CDC), conducts research on environmental health hazards and recommends federal standards for OSHA and for mine safety. The Agency for Toxic Substances and Disease Registry (ATSDR) was created in 1980. Although part of the Department of Health and Human Services, ATSDR is housed at the CDC and has a comprehensive mission with regard to preventing exposure to hazardous substances. These agencies all have comprehensive websites; two other sites relevant to the environment are Toxnet (http://toxnet.nlm.nih.gov) and the Toxics Release Inventory (TRI) (http://www.epa.gov/tri).

POPULATION HEALTH ASSESSMENT

Most people consider themselves members of many different groups. These might include ethnic identifications, age categories, geopolitical constituencies, social classes, or religion adherents. In fact, all these classifications have been used at one time or another to categorize people for the purposes of public health intervention, research, and analysis. In Chapter 3, "Strategies for Entering and Understanding Your Community," various bio-statistical measures that describe events at the population level were presented, including birth rates, death rates, and morbidity rates, along with the major kinds of epidemiological studies used to determine risks and probable causes.

Using rates rather than raw numbers enables the comparison of one group with another to discover differences in health status between and among populations. After differences are found, the next step is to ask why. For example, why is the rate of infant mortality different from one community to another? Among racial and ethnic groups? Between teenagers and adults? Although less easy to discover, it is not very different from asking why a patient has a temperature higher or lower than the average body temperature of the human population, 98.6 degrees Fahrenheit.

Life expectancy and health related quality of life differ among populations within a community, and the capacity of a community to eliminate health disparities and achieve health equity for all is assessed by monitoring rates and trends in those areas in which differences are manifest. Healthy People 2020 has advanced the national agenda from reducing health disparities to eliminating disparities and attaining health equity for all. Health equity is described as follows:

> Health equity entails special efforts to improve the health of those who have experienced social or economic disadvantage. It is a desirable goal/standard that requires 1) a continuous effort focused on elimination of health disparities, including disparities in health care and in the living and working conditions that influence health, and 2) a continuous effort to maintain a desired state of equity after particular health disparities are eliminated. (Healthy People 2020)

Measures to assess the attainment of health for all include tracking of morbidity and mortality rates and chronic health conditions across demographic factors such as race and ethnicity, gender, sexual identity and orientation, disability status, and geographic location (Healthy People 2020). This section contains a discussion not only of the more commonly collected mortality and morbidity rates, but also the behaviors that influence them, the risk factors associated with them, and the high-risk groups in which they are found. The categories chosen for organizing these data are not mutually exclusive. AIDS, for example, is both an infectious and a chronic disease, and certain health behaviors, such as regular exercise, are equally cogent in school age children and adults.

Although addressed here as discrete areas, many health problems are interrelated and multidimensional. Interventions to ameliorate them often must involve biological, behavioral, and environmental factors. For example, problems in behavioral health often accompany disability, the infant-mortality rate is influenced by income level and access to prenatal care, and sexually transmitted infections reflect modal behavioral patterns that characterize subpopulations, such as sex workers or adolescents.

Infectious Diseases

Suggested Activity

Do the following:

- Name the community's five major acute infectious diseases.
- Identify the rates and trends of health care–associated infections.
- Compare local rates for the top five infectious diseases with state and national rates.
- Compare current rates of infectious disease with the previous five and 10 years.
- Note the incidence and prevalence for HIV/AIDS, sexually transmitted infections, and tuberculosis.
- Report epidemics occurring or ongoing in past year, five years, and 10 years.
- Identify populations disproportionately affected by infectious disease.

The World Health Organization (WHO), the CDC, and state boards of health monitor infectious and communicable diseases. Certain infectious diseases are mandated as reportable by federal and state law. These may vary among states and are modified as health problems change. In the past, smallpox was reportable until it was eradicated as a public health problem. Some highly infectious diseases (measles and influenza), or diseases that derive from food or water contamination (salmonella and giardia), result in epidemics. An epidemic traditionally is defined as a greater number of cases than expected, found in a particular place at a particular point in time. This flexible definition affords public health authorities considerable latitude in responding to local-level situations. Tracking and controlling epidemics constitutes a specialized endeavor, and epidemiologists usually are responsible for the initial recommendations for population intervention once their cause and location are determined. Community health nurses, however, may be the first to see these changes and are responsible for reporting them.

The infectious diseases most prevalent in the United States are influenza and pneumonia, and they disproportionately affect children and elders. Over the past two decades, both HIV/AIDS and other sexually transmitted infections have occurred at epidemic rates, with those under 40, gay men, and IV drug abusers disproportionately affected. Most infectious diseases can be prevented through immunization, education, and/or screening.

Chronic Diseases

Suggested Activity

Do the following:

- Cite the mortality and morbidity rates pertaining to the following:
    - Asthma
    - Chronic obstructive pulmonary disease
    - Alzheimer's disease and other dementias
    - Heart disease and stroke
    - Diabetes
    - Chronic kidney disease
    - Cancer
    - Arthritis, osteoporosis and chronic back conditions
- Report the five major noninfectious, chronic diseases reported in the community.
- Identify the differences between local rates and state and national levels.
- Identify the differences between current rates and the previous five and 10 years.
- Describe reasons for the trends and differences.
- Identify populations disproportionately affected by chronic disease.

Valid, reliable, and current data on noninfectious and chronic diseases throughout the world is available through the WHO (http://www.who.int/topics/chronic_diseases). National data are available through the CDC website on Chronic Disease Prevention and Health Promotion (http://www.cdc.gov/chronicdisease). Noninfectious and chronic diseases increasingly are reported at the community level. Much of the data are available at the state and local community health department websites. Additionally, many states and regions have cancer registries where prevalence, if not incidence, data are available. Voluntary health organizations, often national in scope (for example, American Heart Association, American Cancer Society), also are potential sources of morbidity data on noninfectious and chronic diseases such as cardiovascular disease, cancer, chronic pulmonary disease, diabetes, and neuromuscular disease.

The leading causes of death and disability in the United States are coronary heart disease, cancer, and diabetes (CDC, 2010). Alone, stroke, cancer, and heart disease are the cause of more than 50% of annual deaths (Kung, Hoyert, Xu, and Murphy, 2008). Intervention at all three levels of prevention is indicated for chronic diseases, and many are preventable or at least manageable with attention to risk factors such as lack of physical activity, tobacco use, excessive alcohol consumption, and poor nutrition. Because early signs and symptoms often are not recognized, and because health behaviors are related to the most common chronic diseases, intervention strategies at various stages of the disease are critical. With treatment advances, some infectious diseases, such as HIV/AIDS, have become chronic, suggesting new classifications for illness.

Chronic Disability

Suggested Activity

Do the following:

- Cite the rate of physically handicapped or disabled people in the community.
- Report the distribution by age and sex.
- Compare with state, national, and international rates.
- Compare rates over five and 10 years.
- Describe factors that explain trends and differences.

■ Identify disproportionately affected populations.

■ List the percentage of frail elders over 65

Closely linked to the prevalence of chronic disease is the rate of chronic disability in the community. The increasing age of the American population and concomitant musculoskeletal conditions including arthritis, osteoporosis, and chronic back pain are the major causes of disability in the United States. Disabled individuals are more likely to be depressed, obese, hypertensive, unemployed, and psychologically distressed.

Healthy People 2020 identifies the following courses of action:

■ Improving the conditions of daily life

■ Addressing the inequitable distribution of resources among people with disabilities and those without disabilities

■ Expanding the knowledge-base awareness about determinants of health for people with disabilities as three public health goals.

Although chronic disabilities may not be reversed, functional ability and quality of life can be enhanced for the disabled population through public action and policies authorizing parking, wheelchair ramps, curb access, public transportation access, special schools, and facilities. These interventions are a component of the public health infrastructure and just as important as clinical management in ensuring quality of life, ability to function optimally, and productive social relations.

Behavioral and Mental Health

Suggested Activity

Do the following:

- Cite mortality and morbidity rates pertaining to the following behavioral health problems:
    - Depression
    - Domestic violence (child and spouse)
    - Sexual abuse (incest and rape)
    - Suicide
    - Addictive disorder
- Compare these figures with state, national, and international levels.
- Compare these figures with the previous five and 10 years.
- Describe factors explaining the differences.
- Report admission rates for addictive-disorders treatment programs.
- Report discharge rates for alcohol-related illnesses.
- Identify whether homelessness is a problem in the community.
- Identify disproportionately affected populations.

Surveillance of a community's health status also includes determination of various types of behavioral-health problems. The burden of these kinds of disabilities is profoundly under-recognized in this area (Healthy People 2020), yet data are essential for planning appropriate health services, whether ambulatory, residential, or in-patient, and for protective services for victims of abuse and crime. One of the most common causes of disability and disease burden is mental disorders, which results in 25% of years of life lost (WHO, 2011). The suicide rate is a useful indicator of the behavioral/mental health of any population. As the 11th leading cause of death, approximately 30,000 people commit suicide each year (CDC, 2010; NIH, NIMH, 2008; Healthy People 2020). The prevention and recognition of behavioral-health disorders, along with education to eliminate associated social stigma, are necessary to address the pervasive impact they have on the health of all communities.

Maternal, Infant, and Child Health

Suggested Activity

Do the following:

- Cite the community's maternal-, infant-, and child-health statistics, including the following:
  - The neonatal mortality rate
  - The infant mortality rate
  - The maternal mortality rate
- Compare these figures with the previous five and 10 years.
- Compare local, state, national, and international rates.
- Cite explanations for trends and differences.
- Report the most common cause of death for preschoolers.
- Report the most common morbidity in preschoolers.
- Identify populations disproportionately affected in terms of morbidity and mortality, low birth weight, and preterm births.

Suggested Activity

Do the following:

- Cite the percentage of women receiving prenatal and postnatal care.
- Cite the percentage of preschool-age children immunized.
- Cite the percentage of preschool-age children receiving well-child care.
- Report the rate of teenage pregnancy.
- Report the nutritional status of mothers and preschoolers.
- Report the percentage of pregnant mothers who smoke or abuse alcohol or other drugs.
- Identify the populations disproportionately engaging in detrimental health behaviors.

Maternal-child health is designated as one of the topic areas of Healthy People 2020. Significant emphasis is placed on the social and physical determinants of health and the behaviors that promote health, such as early prenatal care, breast-feeding, and smoking and substance-abuse prevention. Traditionally, some of the most commonly used health statistics focus on maternal, infant, and child health as a measure of the well-being of a population. Poverty, access to health care, nutrition, social support, age, and the status of women in the community can all affect pregnancy, childbirth, and maternal and infant survival. As such, crude birth rates and mortality and morbidity data for mothers, infants, and children provide a rough, but meaningful, indication of the health status of a population. Most of the risk to infants occurs in the first weeks of life, and mortality rates for this period have implications for improvements in both the prenatal and postpartum environments. The successful outcome of pregnancy and the ability of an infant to survive through the toddler stage provide strong testimony to the availability and accessibility of maternal-, infant-, and child-health services. Therefore they continue to be used as some of the most significant measures of public health of local, state, national, and international populations.

$$\text{CRUDE BIRTH RATE} = \frac{\text{Total number of live births}}{\text{Total population}} \times 1{,}000$$

$$\text{Neonatal mortality rate} = \frac{\text{Number of deaths under 28 days of age}}{\text{Number of live births}} \times 1{,}000$$

$$\text{Infant mortality rate} = \frac{\text{Number of deaths under 1 year of age}}{\text{Number of live births}} \times 1{,}000$$

$$\text{Maternal mortality rate} = \frac{\text{Number of deaths related to pregnancy and childbirth}}{\text{Number of live births}} \times 10{,}000$$

Morbidity and mortality statistics are most effective in measuring the health of a community when used in conjunction with other kinds of assessment data, such as health linked behavior. In contrast to illness and disease indicators, health indicators may include, for example, the nutritional status of children as reflected in growth and development statistics, the completion rates of high-school students, immunization rates, and well-child care. Federal guidelines recommend that children be immunized by the age of 3 years for the following: diphtheria, pertussis and tetanus; measles, mumps and rubella; polio; varicella; hepatitis A; hepatitis B; pneumococcal pneumonia; and haemophilus influenzae type B.

Early and Middle Childhood Health

Suggested Activity

Do the following:

- Cite leading causes of morbidity and mortality.
- Report nutritional status.
- Cite statistics on vision and hearing.
- Report growth and development status.
- Report performance on national achievement tests.
- Cite the proportion of the population that is adequately immunized.
- Cite the proportion of the population receiving routine well-child care.
- Cite the proportion of the population receiving routine dental care.
- Describe any problems associated with violence in this population.
- Report the incidence of childhood suicides in the past five years.
- Identify populations disproportionately affected by high morbidity, mortality, or detrimental health behavior.

Early childhood is birth to age 8; middle childhood is ages 6 to 12 (Healthy People 2020). According the Healthy People 2020, these stages of childhood have had little focus in the past. Yet they are recognized to have specific developmental tasks that are important to healthy development, as well as risk factors such as asthma, obesity, dental caries, maltreatment, and developmental and behavioral disorders. The Healthy People 2020 public health agenda seeks to better understand and plan for the needs of this population, including supportive environments, access to high-quality health care, and knowledgeable and nurturing families. Schools and recreational facilities are two locations for educating children and their families about health promotion as well as disease prevention and management.

Adolescent Health

Suggested Activity

Do the following:

- Cite leading causes of morbidity and mortality in adolescents.
- Cite nutritional status.
- Cite performance on national achievement tests.
- Report the proportion of the population that is adequately immunized.
- Report the proportion of the population receiving routine health care.
- Report the proportion of the population receiving routine dental care.
- Report the proportion of the population using alcohol and/or drugs.
- Report the rate and types of violence in the population.
- Report the incidence of adolescent suicides in the past five years.
- Identify populations disproportionately affected by high morbidity, mortality, or detrimental health behavior.

A new topic of Healthy People 2020 is adolescent health. Included are those persons who are typical adolescents, ages 10 to 19, and young adults ages 20 to 24, who together make up 21% of the U.S. population. Because both healthy lifestyle patterns and risky behaviors are established during this time, the goal of Healthy People 2020 is to "improve the healthy development, health, safety, and well-being of adolescents and young adults." Adolescents have been shown to be amenable to socially supported health promotion programs such as pregnancy, violence, and delinquency-prevention programs. With increased ethnic diversity in the U.S. population, however, the tailoring of these programs to be culturally informed remains a public health challenge.

Older Adult Health

Suggested Activity

Do the following:

- Cite leading causes of morbidity and mortality in the older-adult population.
- Report the nutritional status of the older-adult population.
- Cite the proportion of the older-adult population that is adequately immunized.
- Report the proportion of the older-adult population receiving routine health care.
- Cite the proportion of the older-adult population receiving routine dental care.
- Cite the proportion of older adults using alcohol or drugs.
- Identify the rate and type of older-adult abuse and neglect in the community.
- Report the incidence of older-adult suicides in the past five years.
- Identify disproportionately affected populations in terms of high morbidity, mortality, or detrimental health behavior.

It is well-known that older adults constitute the fastest-growing age group not only in the United States but worldwide (U.S. Census, 2008; WHO, 2011). The increase in life expectancy is a public health success, and it brings opportunities for increased participation of older persons in society. Population-aging also brings an increased risk for chronic disease such as diabetes, arthritis, dementia, and congestive heart failure with associated disabilities and social marginalization. Injury prevention is critical for older persons, particularly building healthy environments and lifestyle behaviors to prevent falls—the leading unintentional injury cause of death for older adults (WHO, 2004).

With chronic illness often comes an associated need for assistance. Most older adults are cared for by family members or someone in their own home. With an estimated one to two million older adults being injured or abused by a caregiver (National Research Council, 2003), awareness and development of culturally informed caregiver-education and abuse-prevention programs is critical (Institute of Medicine, 2008). It is important to determine what social activities, health prevention and promotion programs, and other services are available and accessible to older persons in the community. A health assessment should include the identification of hidden populations of elders in the community, such as undocumented older persons living with their immigrant children.

Lesbian, Gay, Bisexual, and Transgender (LGBT) Health

Suggested Activity

Do the following:

- Cite leading causes of morbidity and mortality in the LGBT population.
- Cite the proportion of the LGBT population receiving routine health care.
- Report the proportion of the LGBT population receiving routine dental care.
- Report the proportion of the LGBT population using alcohol or drugs.
- Identify whether violence is a problem in the LGBT population.
- Report the incidence of LGBT suicides in the past five years.

The health status of the lesbian, gay, bisexual, and transgendered population is a new topic area in Healthy People 2020. Identified as a population that suffers high rates of stigma, violence, discrimination, human-rights violations, and health disparities, LGBT populations are more likely to be obese or overweight; use tobacco, alcohol, and other drugs; and, as youth, attempt suicide and be homeless (Healthy People 2020). As background to an effective community health assessment, consider the following key LGBT issues identified by Healthy People 2020:

■ Prevention of violence and homicide toward the LGB and especially the transgender population.

■ Gathering of nationally representative data on LGBT Americans

■ Resiliency of LGBT communities

■ LGBT parenting issues throughout the life course

■ Elder health and well-being

■ Exploration of sexual/gender identity among youth

■ Need for a LGBT wellness model

■ Recognition of transgender health needs as medically necessary

Occupational Safety and Health

Suggested Activity

Do the following:

■ List the most common health problems found in the adult workforce.

■ Report rate of absenteeism in the adult workforce.

■ List the most common reasons cited for absenteeism.

■ Report percentage of worker population receiving a routine physical examination.

■ Report percentage of the workforce engaging in a routine exercise program.

■ Identify occupational groups disproportionately characterized by health problems, absenteeism, and negative health behaviors.

The health of our adult workforce is another measure of the ability of a population to meet the challenges of its environment. The development of health problems or a decrease in performance levels has serious implications for the economy of the community. Many causes of disability are related to the aging of the workforce population as well as the work itself and to working conditions, low back pain and carpal-tunnel syndrome being two common examples. In addition, alcohol- and drug-related problems, violence, and abuse often are identified and addressed in work settings that have comprehensive health programs. The workplace is an ideal setting for addressing negative health behaviors and for promoting healthy behavior.

Population Health Behaviors

Suggested Activity

Do the following:

- Cite the percentage of the population exhibiting the following:
  - Satisfaction with engagement in social activities, programs, and relationships
  - An active exercise program
  - A smokeless lifestyle
  - Satisfaction with quality of life
- Cite the percentage of the population exhibiting the following detrimental health behaviors:
  - Tobacco-smoking
  - Illicit drug use
  - Excessive alcohol use
  - Overeating or poor eating habits
  - Inadequate physical activity
- Indicate the percentage of the population exhibiting detrimental health characteristics such as hypertension, high cholesterol, and obesity.
- Identify populations disproportionately exhibiting these behaviors.

Health behaviors can be precursors to wellness or illness, and often serve to place members of the population in an at-risk group. The CDC has standardized a survey used by all states since 1994 that is reported in the Behavioral Risk Factor Surveillance System, with state-level data provided. Other sources of these data may include the Healthy People 2020 website and surveys by local organizations on smoking, substance abuse, and sexual behavior. Unhealthy behavior traditionally has been a target for nursing intervention and personal health services. Its usefulness in community health practice, however, lies equally, if not more, in identifying the disparities among populations and interpreting those disparities in health behavior *vis-à-vis* community determinants.

The various dimensions of a population-based health assessment presented thus far provide just a sampling of the unlimited range of criteria that can be used to evaluate the health of a population. Depending on the community, certain circumstances or problems may require more detailed information or even different assessment criteria. It is always preferable, however, to make the best possible use of existing data.

Statistics and other health status indicators can provide powerful information about the relative health status of a population and convincing evidence about health disparities and the need to take public health action. There are, however, several caveats to remember in their use. As mentioned in Chapter 3, rates must be adjusted or standardized according to demographic characteristics and the size of the community. The morbidity and mortality rates in a small community may be deceptive when compared to a large community, and they must be viewed over a longer time sequence to compensate for the small numbers. Most important, the data must be accurate and systematically collected. Death-registry data generally are more reliable than data from birth registries, although one cannot always depend on the accuracy of the recorded cause of death. Certainly, not all births are registered and not all occurrences of a disease are reported, particularly for stigmatized health problems such as sexually transmitted infections, psychiatric problems, and alcohol abuse.

HEALTH CARE ORGANIZATION ASSESSMENT

Like education, family, work, recreation, and other human institutions, the pursuit of health has a set of specialized activities, roles, norms, and values in society. The third component of the community health assessment is an investigation of health and health care as a social institution and an evaluation of its capacity to create a healthy community. All societies have ideological belief and value systems as well as specialized personnel and rituals designed not only to care for the sick (McElroy and Townsend, 2004), but also to promote the health of people in communities.

PREVENTION AND HEALTH PROMOTION

A healthy community is one that is meeting the goals of Healthy People 2020. Thus, the focus of the public health infrastructure includes economic stability, educational opportunity, a safe and clean environment, robust community institutions, and universal citizen participation. As a discipline and profession, public health has endorsed prevention and health promotion as its principal methods for achieving health. Therefore, a health assessment must include an evaluation of the community's infrastructure for prevention as a fundamental aspect of the cultural capital of the community. There are three levels of prevention, each of which corresponds to a set of health programs and personnel that make up the cultural capital for public health promotion:

- **Primary prevention:** The goal of primary prevention is to reduce the occurrence of illness and disability in the community and to increase health and well-being. Primary prevention strategies for a community's health presuppose a healthy population and ordinarily include clean air, soil, and water; good sanitation; adequate nutrition; and safe physical and social environments in which to live, work, and play. The direct correlation between the standard of living and health status of a community is a commonly accepted axiom of public health, and many of our most intractable public health problems historically are correlated with poverty (Heymann, Hertzman, Barer, and Evans, 2006; Reagan and Salsberry, 2005). Thus, the effectiveness of primary prevention is measured by the quality of the physical and social environment and community wide access to health and health care as well as by the traditional mortality (death) and morbidity (illness) statistics. The range of primary prevention interventions, therefore, could include urban gardens, early-parenting programs, installation of traffic lights at busy intersections, nutrition-education programs in primary schools, and sanitary inspections in restaurants.

■ **Secondary prevention:** The goal of secondary prevention is to diagnose and treat public health problems as early as possible and to restore a complete state of health in the shortest possible time. Building community capacity for secondary prevention is accomplished through identifying health risks and problems as well as timely intervention. Primary care clinics, weight-reduction and smoking-cessation programs, river cleanup, driver-safety programs for traffic-law offenders, razing dangerous vacant buildings, and shelters for the homeless all qualify as examples of secondary prevention. Secondary prevention presupposes the ability to restore the health and abilities of the community and its residents. Similar to primary prevention action, secondary-prevention action can be measured by mortality and morbidity rates, but other measures such as response time of intervention, the proportion of populations screened for specific health risks, and the affordability and accessibility of health and social services provide additional useful indicators. Police departments, fire departments, and shelters for victims of domestic violence are examples of cultural capital for secondary prevention.

■ **Tertiary prevention:** The goal of tertiary prevention in public health is to provide the highest quality of life for those persons and segments of the community who have experienced severe trauma or disease, are disabled, or are chronically or terminally ill. Home care services, hospitals, rehabilitation centers, long term–care facilities, and hospice are examples of community cultural capital designated for tertiary prevention. With the exception of public hospitals and clinics typically located in major urban centers, the responsibility of public health in tertiary prevention ordinarily is ensuring the safety and supportiveness of tertiary prevention facilities. This could include safe egress of institutionalized residents in a fire; laws pertaining to patient abuse; regulations governing cleanliness, food services, and staff ratios in long term–care facilities; and certification of home health agencies. An outstanding example of tertiary prevention in the United States is the Americans with Disabilities Act, which mandates the provision of access to persons with disabilities.

Finally while public health departments usually focus on system level interventions, some kinds of personal health services qualify as public health prevention services because they reduce risk or prevent widespread disease and disability. Such programs not only improve the health of the community but also reduce the costs of expensive hospitalizations and medical care. Well-child care, flu immunization programs for health care workers, home safety installations for elders, school health services, prenatal clinics, hypertension monitoring, early detection screening for prostate cancer, and testing for HIV/AIDS are just a few examples.

All three levels of prevention constitute public health action, and often are found in a single initiative. Public education for disaster readiness, for example, may be classified as primary prevention. Readiness programs also include immediate and restorative treatment, such as shelters and access to food and potable water (secondary prevention) and enlistment of hospitals for emergency and acute care of the seriously injured and mental-health programs for those who have lost a family member or suffer from disaster related post-traumatic stress disorder (PTSD) (tertiary prevention). The integration of programs that support intervention at all three levels of prevention is ideal, not only for optimal outcomes, but also for cost-effectiveness.

Public Health Services: Health Care Institutions

Suggested Activity

Do the following:

- Describe the health care institutions responsible for monitoring and promoting the health of the public.
- Describe the process for establishing health care policies in the community.

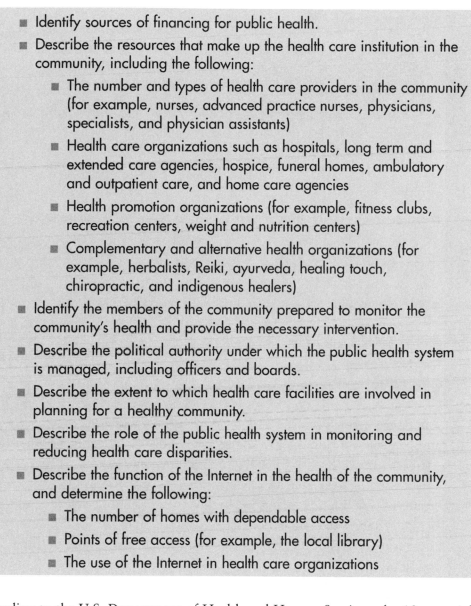

- Identify sources of financing for public health.
- Describe the resources that make up the health care institution in the community, including the following:
    - The number and types of health care providers in the community (for example, nurses, advanced practice nurses, physicians, specialists, and physician assistants)
    - Health care organizations such as hospitals, long term and extended care agencies, hospice, funeral homes, ambulatory and outpatient care, and home care agencies
    - Health promotion organizations (for example, fitness clubs, recreation centers, weight and nutrition centers)
    - Complementary and alternative health organizations (for example, herbalists, Reiki, ayurveda, healing touch, chiropractic, and indigenous healers)
- Identify the members of the community prepared to monitor the community's health and provide the necessary intervention.
- Describe the political authority under which the public health system is managed, including officers and boards.
- Describe the extent to which health care facilities are involved in planning for a healthy community.
- Describe the role of the public health system in monitoring and reducing health care disparities.
- Describe the function of the Internet in the health of the community, and determine the following:
    - The number of homes with dependable access
    - Points of free access (for example, the local library)
    - The use of the Internet in health care organizations

According to the U.S. Department of Health and Human Services, the 10 essential services to guide the responsibilities of the public health infrastructure are as follows (Centers for Disease Control and Prevention, 2010):

- Monitor health status to identify and solve community health problems

- Diagnose and investigate health problems and health hazards in the community

- Inform, educate, and empower people about health issues

- Mobilize community partnerships and action to identify and solve health problems

- Develop policies and plans that support individual and community health efforts

- Enforce laws and regulations that protect health and ensure safety

- Link people to needed personal health services and assure the provision of health care when otherwise unavailable

- Assure a competent public and personal health care workforce

- Evaluate effectiveness, accessibility, and quality of personal and population-based health services

- Research for new insights and innovative solutions to health problems

Although personal health services in the United States are considered to be the most sophisticated in the world, the limitations of our public health system are increasingly evidenced by population health indicators that are inconsistent with the continuing rise in health care costs. In its charge to protect and promote the health of communities, managing both urgent and chronic threats, our public health system is the foundation for successful population-health outcomes. The three components of the public health infrastructure required to fulfill the essential public health services are as follows (Healthy People 2020):

- A capable and qualified workforce

- Up-to-date data and information systems

- Agencies capable of assessing and responding to community health needs

THE PUBLIC HEALTH WORKFORCE

Public health draws from an interdisciplinary workforce from fields such as medicine, public health, nursing, epidemiology, and sanitation. In 2003, the Quad Council of Public Health Nursing Organizations identified public health nursing competencies for the generalist and specialist that included the following skills:

- Analytic assessment

- Policy development/program planning

- Communication

- Cultural competency

- Community dimensions of practice

- Basic public health sciences

- Financial planning and management

- Leadership and systems thinking

Similarly, in 2010, the Council on Linkages between Academia and Public Health Practice approved core competencies for public health professionals at three levels: entry, management and/or supervisory responsibilities, and senior managers and/or leaders (Public Health Foundation, 2010). These competencies are in the same areas as those in the preceding list.

Healthy People 2020 includes objectives to do the following:

- Incorporate the core competencies for public health professionals into job descriptions and performance evaluations.

- Increase continuing education based on the competencies.

- Increase the proportion of Council on Education for Public Health (CEPH)–accredited schools of public health and schools of nursing.

- Increase the proportion of four-year colleges and universities and two-year colleges that offer public health or associated programs.

INFORMATION SYSTEMS

An ongoing challenge is to link health related agencies in such a way that health information systems can be organized into integrated systems. One effort to systematize information and communication was realized with the adoption by most states of common health status indicators to gauge community health status and the use of technology to facilitate the description, tracking, and comparing of health indicators.

The goals of Healthy People 2020 include the following:

- Increasing the national data available for all major population groups

- Increasing the proportion of objectives that are tracked at the national level every three years

- Accelerating the speed with which national data are released at the end of data collection

- Increase the number of states recording births and deaths using standard certificates of birth

PUBLIC HEALTH AGENCIES

Not surprisingly, there is great variation among communities in the kind and breadth of their health infrastructures and the services they provide. Also, communities vary with regard to the resources obtainable to address community health problems. One of the great ironies in public health practice is that the communities with the most problems usually have the fewest resources. As revealed in the preceding sections, these health disparities are detectable in both the populations and the environments of communities.

Health Departments

In the United States and increasingly throughout the world, the responsibilities for health consist of a complex organization of proprietary (for-profit), voluntary (non-profit), and public (governmental) agencies that together constitute an increasingly entrepreneurial health care system. Most incorporated or geopolitically designated communities—townships, municipalities, and counties—have a health department as part of their government charters. Health departments are those organizations ordinarily provided by government statute to monitor and improve the health of the public and the environments in which they live. Typically, they are conterminous with geopolitical boundaries and organized in a pyramid of administrative accountability by town or city, county, state, and nation. Historically, physician commissioners have headed health departments, but this has changed dramatically within the past few decades as community health nurses have been increasingly tapped for these leadership posts.

Health departments vary greatly in their range of responsibilities, but most include both environmental and population health services. Usually, they are accountable for the bulk of primary prevention initiatives: public health education, preparedness, communicable disease prevention, maternal-child–health promotion, environmental protection, sanitation, inspection of food and health industries, emission standards, and the preparation of vital statistics, to name just a few. Depending on the community, they may be responsible for some secondary- and tertiary prevention programs, such as control of communicable diseases and direct care services to underserved populations in the form of primary care centers, chronic disease management, and acute care in public hospitals. Monitoring health disparities and health equity has been added to the responsibilities of more and more health departments across the nation.

Health departments usually are overseen or advised by boards of health. The manner in which board members are selected (appointment or election), the length of their terms in office, and the professional criteria for their selection varies with the local governance structure, as does their role to direct or advise the health department. Their status and position within the wider community and their philosophies on health care will strongly influence the contributions of individual members. In small communities, it is not unusual for many of the board members to have little or no background in health sciences or health practice. This provides an opportunity for nurses to educate and advise politicians and other board members about the value of public health services for promoting and sustaining healthy communities and reducing the tax burden on the residents.

Personal Health Care Agencies

Health departments work with local hospitals, extended care facilities, home-health and ambulatory services such as clinics, and private practices in ensuring the health of a community. Hospitals, for example, often are viewed as providing only secondary and tertiary services, but hospital blood banks and disaster preparedness programs constitute a critical component of the community's readiness for emergencies. Hospital records provide important data that can be used by epidemiologists to detect and explain various public health problems. More recently, hospitals have expanded their community responsibilities to play an important role in maintaining the health of uninsured populations through community health education programs such as cardiac-health programs that help individuals extend the years and quality of healthy life. By law, all not-for-profit hospitals are required to provide evidence of the extent and nature of the benefit they provide for their surrounding communities to qualify for tax exempt status.

Health Planning Agencies

Most communities have a formal organization officially appointed to coordinate and plan the continued health of the population and environment. In 1946, the federal government launched its first health planning initiative with the Hill-Burton Hospital Survey and Construction Act. This act provided funds to assist states in financing hospital construction. States were required to formulate a plan for the organization of hospitals and other facilities based on the existing facilities and utilization data. In 1962, federal funding became available for statewide health planning activities. In 1966, Public Law 89–749, the Comprehensive Health Planning and Community Health Service Amendments, authorized health planning on a state and regional basis. As a result, federally mandated health-planning agencies have been established to ensure that some pressing needs are not ignored while excesses exist in other areas. Such agencies are responsible not only for coordinating and developing local health services, but also for articulating health planning with other kinds of community planning.

PUBLIC HEALTH FINANCING

Traditionally, health departments were supported almost exclusively through state and local public funding from tax revenues, and they provided a limited range of services to residents at minimum or no charge. Now, however, it is not unusual to have at least part of the department's revenue based in fee-for-service activities charged to Medicare and Medicaid funds. The existence of health departments is a clear statement that health is a public responsibility. Unfortunately, because they depend on public funds, health departments are highly sensitive to the vagaries of partisan politics. Programs that receive full support in one party's term may be put on the back shelf as another political party takes office. In addition, when fiscal crises arise, public health programs may be sacrificed if they are not "entitlement" programs, such as Medicare or Medicaid.

In the highly entrepreneurial U.S. health care system, an assessment of financial resources is very revealing. There are many possible sources from which facilities derive their revenues, such as private insurers, public insurers, fee-for-service models, charity, and pre-paid health care plans. Another approach to financing is to look at the financial resources available to residents, such as self-pay, health insurance, health maintenance organizations, charity (formal and informal), public assistance, or government insurance (for example, Medicaid and Medicare). In many communities, care of the medically indigent has fallen to the health department and public hospitals. Because all services must be paid by someone, the cost of providing care to non-insured persons ultimately is assumed by the taxpayer. In assessing the public health infrastructure, it is important to identify health programs and activities that are publicly supported, without charge or at a nominal charge to qualified residents. These could include school physicals, dental hygiene, immunizations and prenatal care provided by the health department, as well as those services provided by funds raised by voluntary associations or other community groups. The source and method of reimbursement for health services will profoundly affect the distribution, quality, and range of services provided. Despite acclamation for the value of prevention and early detection, unless such activities are reimbursed or supported in some manner, they will continue to be omitted in the range of services provided to communities.

Many uninsured individuals and families have no consistent provider of primary care and often do not receive primary and secondary services. Because we do not leave the sick or injured to die on the steps of a hospital, such uninsured individuals and families use health care services in the most expensive tertiary venues (emergency departments and hospitals) for conditions that might have been prevented if they had been seen in a primary care clinic. The Affordable Care and Patient Protection Act passed in 2010 is the nation's attempt to increase access to basic health care services and reign in escalating health care costs. This health care reform is a response to the lack of accountability among all three components of the health care triangle: patients, providers, and third party payers. Patients have failed, as a group, to engage in healthier lifestyles; many providers have opportunistically provided unnecessary and excessive services; and insurers have procrastinated in developing reimbursement models that increase the use of preventive services and reduce reliance on expensive acute care. Within the past decade, the national public health system has taken the lead through Medicare (Centers for Medicare and Medicaid Services) by injecting accountability into the system through incentives, such as pay-for-performance formulas, and penalties, such as denials of reimbursement for hospital-acquired conditions and for readmissions to the hospital within 30 days of discharge.

Health Values and Beliefs

Suggested Activity

Do the following:

- Identify the common beliefs held by local populations about the cause, prevention, and treatment of public health problems.
- Describe common health and health care customs within the community
- List health and health care traditions within the community.
- Describe the various opinions about what constitutes a healthy community.
- Identify three public health interventions that have generated community conflict.
- Identify the age considered to be a "natural" age at which to die.
- Describe the variation in health care values and beliefs present in this community.

The decisions made by health departments and boards of health are heavily influenced by local beliefs and values about public health. Although beliefs about health are not uniformly held or acted upon by all members of a society, it is nevertheless possible to identify a broad range of health ideas, values, and practices that guide and shape the public health infrastructure of a community. Almost all culture groups have theories of causation that guide disease prevention in the absence of scientific explanation. For example, the virus theory of infectious disease explains why individuals contract influenza, but it does not explain why some persons acquire the disease and others do not, even though their exposure was the same. Another example is the commonly held belief that childhood immunizations will cause autism, leading some parents to refuse to allow their children to be immunized.

The endorsement of public services requires, minimally, that people believe the potential for a public health problem exists, and that the problem is amenable to public health intervention. Some members of the community may view violence in schools as a singular, pathological event rather than as an indication of widespread adolescent disenfranchisement. Others may view health disparities as just part of the natural order of society rather than as a symptom of an unhealthy and unjust society. Even the most homogenous communities report a lack of agreement on what distinguishes a public health problem from a personal health problem. The variation in meanings that specific health conditions and behaviors hold for different groups must be considered in planning for the public's health. A lack of understanding between health professionals and the lay public on the definition of a public health problem and the appropriate prevention and treatment can have a profound effect on the success of efforts to build community capacity and ameliorate the problem.

INDIGENOUS AND ALTERNATIVE HEALTH SYSTEMS

Finally, when assessing the public health infrastructure of a community, it would be inaccurate to assume that only one health system is operative, and that people do not avail themselves of alternatives to the biomedical system of Western medicine. Rather than making assumptions, it is better simply to ask, how do people in this community protect their health? How do they make their community a healthier place? The answers to such questions can reveal indigenous local health care institutions and the degree to which they are embedded in local culture and connected with other health care institutions.

Most populations pursue all the health resources available to them. If, for instance, two distinct systems are in place, it is common for both to be used (Whitaker, 2003). Anthropologists have labeled this "medical pluralism." Given the large populations of ethnically diverse and immigrant groups in many communities, it is incumbent upon community practitioners to know the range of the health care infrastructure available within them. By far, the greatest share of personal health care in any society takes place in the home, where methods of caring and remedies have passed through families over generations.

Most communities have alternative and complementary institutions and providers who offer health care services such as healing touch, Reiki, herbs, ayurveda, meditation, yoga, homeopathy, acupuncture, and nutrition-based practices. In some communities, these systems are less visible but provide the range of primary, secondary, and tertiary prevention in a well-organized, internally consistent system well-known to the community members. Good examples are the *espiritismo* centers found in significant numbers in areas where Cuban and/or Puerto Rican populations reside. These centers usually are located in private homes, where services are provided in the context of group gatherings that have social as well as health functions.

There are several important reasons to acknowledge the presence of complementary and alternative health resources operating in any given community:

- Much can be learned from these traditional modalities, such as the heavy reliance on group and community support as a vehicle for dealing with health problems. The power of group reinforcement, for example, is now being realized in the treatment of substance abuse, diabetes, cancer, obesity, and many other patient and family problems.

- The behavioral norms of subgroups in a community that, at first, may seem odd to outsiders often are rooted in social and/or religious beliefs that have significant local importance in public health. Disregarding or disparaging them can be costly in terms of effectiveness in building community capacity.

- By knowing the logic of complementary and alternative systems, it is possible to place scientific public health practice in a framework that may be more acceptable to community residents. For example, a program for child health and expanding prenatal care in a particular ethnic group must take into account norms regarding male and female role fulfillment, age-appropriate sexual behavior, and family structure, as well as the beliefs and practices associated with successful pregnancy and subsequent parenting. Not every client or patient will express the full range of cultural norms regarding pregnancy and childbirth. It is nonetheless important to understand and accept diverse beliefs and practices.

- The leaders of such complementary and alternative systems are usually charismatic individuals whose local power can be tapped by community practitioners for public health initiatives.

6

LAYING THE FOUNDATION FOR A HEALTHY COMMUNITY AGENDA

Like the Healthy People agenda, a healthy community agenda is a strategic plan, complete with goals, objectives, vision, mission, values, and tactics, that permits us to get things done in a disciplined manner, follow a course of action, and mobilize material and social resources. To be effective, it must be based on knowledge of the community's culture and achieved in partnership with community stakeholders. In this chapter, you learn how to use cultural information to guide all aspects of strategic health planning.

CHAPTER 6 OBJECTIVES

■ Determine the groundwork necessary to develop a strategic plan for a healthy community.

■ Understand the historical and contemporary importance of planning in public health.

■ Compare culture based planning with resource-based and population-based planning.

■ Develop a healthy community agenda, including culturally informed overarching goals, vision, mission, values, measurable objectives, and strategies.

■ Create an effective constituency grounded in community culture.

■ Appraise the effectiveness of strategic planning for creating healthy and sustainable communities.

THE FUTURE IS NOW

Managing the future is an ethical as well as an operational imperative in community health practice. The public health programs that communities have in place today are based on the predictions and plans that were made five, 10, or 20 years ago. Similarly, what happens to our children and grandchildren, and the communities in which they will live, depends on the predictions and plans we make today for 2020, 2030, and 2040. In the day-to-day work of community practice, however, there are so many issues and concerns that require our attention and effort that it is easy to become distracted from our primary mission: to promote and sustain the health of our community. A healthy community agenda is not just a collection of initiatives to resolve particular community problems or issues. It is a thoughtful, comprehensive, and strategic plan, created in partnership with residents, to guide the work we do and the resources we use in shaping the community's future.

The ultimate goal of public health practice is a healthy community. The definitive strategy for public health practice is to work with and through community leaders and groups to enhance community capacity. Finally, you know from previous chapters that a community's health is not simply the aggregate of the health status of its citizens, but rather a physical, economic, and social infrastructure with the capacity to fulfill the overarching goals of Healthy People 2020:

- Attain high-quality, longer lives free of preventable disease, disability, injury, and premature death.

- Achieve health equity, eliminate disparities, and improve the health of all groups.

- Create social and physical environments that promote good health for all.

- Promote quality of life, healthy development, and healthy behaviors across all life stages.

WHY IS PLANNING SO IMPORTANT IN COMMUNITY HEALTH PRACTICE?

Community health practice is necessarily future-oriented. A thoughtful, informed design for the future helps communities effectively manage rather than react to the changes in the physical and social environments that will likely take place over the ensuing decades. Health departments in cities and states across the country, for example, are giving special consideration to the future impact of global warming on their communities. Some of the anticipated effects of climate change that will be especially burdensome for the urban poor, older adults, and those with chronic illness include water and air pollution, which will cause exposure to ozone and result in the following:

- Allergies and other respiratory illnesses

- Direct thermal injury from intense heat

- Extreme weather events resulting in injury and exposure to infectious and vector-borne diseases

The Katrina hurricane and ensuing floods, the tsunamis in Southeast Asia and Japan, the earthquakes in Haiti and Chile, and anthrax, 9/11, and H1N1—all are examples of unpredicted events and various levels of preparedness. They have sensitized public health departments across the nation to the importance of readiness and generated a new set of objectives for Healthy People 2020 focused on preventing, preparing for, responding to, and recovering from future assaults on our communities. The success of response and the resilience to manage such events depend on the extent to which a healthy community agenda has created an engaged and informed citizenry, social interconnectedness, government and private-sector collaboration, and a health care infrastructure that is in a constant state of readiness.

Dramatic changes in the social environments of communities, including industry closures, job loss, housing foreclosures, and population shifts, also can catch communities unaware, with some negative results that, in hindsight, might have been avoided.

Iowa has been the destination of a variety of human migrations—from Mexico, the Sudan, and eastern European countries. No one, however, would have predicted a migration of families from Chicago, where urban renewal and gentrification resulted in the razing of high-rise public housing (Keene, Padilla, and Geronimus, 2010). Notwithstanding the decaying condition of the public housing they left, as well as the associated crime and violence, the displaced Chicagoans lamented the loss of family and friends and the social support they felt in their previous dwellings. Motivated by the pursuit of "peace and quiet," affordable housing, land room, and better schools for their children, they had great expectations of their new homes in Iowa, but they soon found themselves segregated by a community unfamiliar with the urban, African-American culture they brought with them. The introduction of culturally different young families created a challenge for Iowa-based schoolteachers, health care providers, and law-enforcement officials as they tried to interpret and understand the urban life ways of this group. They were caught without a community wide plan for embracing these new members and integrating them into community life. Instead, the existing Iowan community felt "invaded," while the Chicagoans felt "isolated" in a community where occasional gestures of welcome could not compensate for the perceived racial profiling.

HEALTH PLANNING: AS IT WAS, IS, AND CAN BE

To fully understand both the problems and possibilities of contemporary public health and the significance of cultural information in creating a healthy and sustainable future, it is useful to review the evolution of health planning in the United States.

RESOURCE-BASED PLANNING

Despite the original purpose of the boards of health that first appeared in 19th-century England to promote and protect the health of their communities (Gelbach, 2005), health planning in the United States has focused almost exclusively on building health facilities and services—that is, the "bricks and mortar" of health *care*. Hospitals, visiting-nurse agencies, rehabilitation centers, skilled-nursing facilities, mental-health programs, and so on were established in relation to the demand for services. This resource-based planning used the experience of these various health care organizations to anticipate and organize health services. Its underlying strategy was to adjust the existing services to the individuals and families who currently used them. If a home health agency were used to capacity, more nursing staff would be employed or another agency would be opened. Similarly, if a hospital pediatric unit were underutilized, it would be closed or reduced in size.

Managing demand emphasizes the treatment of health problems rather than the prevention of illness and the promotion of health. In resource-based planning, promoting the health of populations and communities to control cost is not a high priority. Nor is there a great emphasis on reducing disparities or controlling excesses. In response to escalating costs of health care, regional models for health resource management began to appear that attempted to link resources and demands with population size and health needs (White, 1973). Primary health care services, for example, which address common but comparatively minor health problems, would be provided in a decentralized model and serve small populations of 1,000 to 25,000. Secondary health facilities (such as community hospitals, extended care facilities, rehabilitation services, and home health care) addressing more serious but common problems would require a population of 25,000 to several hundred thousand to generate a definable demand. Finally, tertiary health care would warrant a population of 500,000 to several million to justify the presence of technologically sophisticated and costly services.

Such models for health care service delivery based on community level services inspired the National Health Planning Resources and Development Act of 1974 (Public Law 93–641), which established 205 local health systems agencies (HSAs) throughout the United States. Each HSA was accountable for planning the organization of health personnel, facilities, and services in designated districts based on a mandated health status profile (in most cases, a health *problem* profile) that must be used to formulate a five-year health systems plan and an annual implementation plan. Public Law 93–641 was supposed to address issues of community prevention and intermediate care, equal access, quality of care, cost, public and private-sector collaboration, and the maldistribution of services along with uncontrolled hospital-cost inflation. The results, however, were sufficiently disappointing to lead to the institution of diagnosis-related groups (DRGs) in 1983 to control hospital stays and, in 2010, the Patient Protection and Affordable Care Act to ensure access and reduce cost.

POPULATION-BASED PLANNING

Although the regional planning efforts of the 1970s did not come to fruition, they paved the way for population-based planning. In the 1970s, a growing sensitivity to consistently at-risk populations shifted our attention away from health resources and individuals who use them. By focusing on populations rather than just patients, health planning efforts began to emphasize risk factors and unmet needs rather than illness and resources. Unlike resource-based planning, which emphasizes care for the sick, population-based planning strives to reduce risk through health promotion. The cost-containment strategy consists of primary prevention, health maintenance, early detection, primary care, and the engagement of other social services including education, recreation, and housing. Based squarely in the science of epidemiology, there are four basic steps to population-based planning:

1. Health problems are identified and prioritized, and the population is subdivided according to distinct health needs (for example, women, school children, elders, the homeless).

2. Risk factors for each problem are identified through a review of the literature, and at-risk or target populations are determined.

3. Interventions needed to reduce or eliminate the problem are formulated.

4. The existing resources are compared with those needed to resolve the problem, and the gaps between them (unmet needs) are designated as essential services that are incorporated in the community health plan.

In population-based planning, we initially ignore existing resources and start with the populations' health problems. We concentrate on what makes people unhealthy or vulnerable. Methods of resolving health problems are not limited to medical intervention or personal health services but include social marketing, policy development, environmental modification, public education, and community awareness. Population-based planning exposes the deficiencies and inequities in health care by drawing attention to those groups consistently at risk, often referred to as *vulnerable populations*: pregnant women, smokers, the overweight, elders living alone without family close by, and the underserved (for example, the poor, homeless, or specific ethnic groups).

Consider the following example to compare resource-based and population-based planning: If epidemiological evidence in an urban community revealed a steadily increasing rate of low-birth-weight infants, the resource-based plan would expand the neonatal intensive care unit and recruit specialized staff. In contrast, the population-based approach would first determine the risk factors and risk groups associated with this problem and, depending on the risk factors (for example, economic, genetic, nutritional, occupational, or educational), formulate a strategy for risk reduction. This might include contraception and family planning, smoking cessation, prenatal counseling and monitoring, nutrition programs, and/or workplace-improvement regulation.

By attending to unmet needs, instead of demand and utilization, population-based planning holds greater promise for preventing—rather than treating—health problems. It is, nevertheless, a deficit model focusing on health problems (such as asthma, obesity, coronary heart disease, crime victimization, traffic accidents). Unhealthy behaviors are treated much like diseases, amenable to interventions such as teaching, reducing alcohol consumption, exercise programs, or special diets. Paradoxically, many of these risks are reframed as individual lifestyle choices rather than problems embedded in the socio-cultural matrix of community life. The population-based approach assumes that the public's health could be improved greatly if individuals would engage in healthier behaviors.

Finally, because of its problem-specific orientation, the population-based method often yields a categorical approach in which a healthy community agenda is composed of several separately funded and operated programs, such as programs devoted to offering health care for women and children, HIV/AIDS, disaster preparedness, lead paint, communicable disease management, and such. There are many problems with categorical funding, not least of which is that we often fail to see how health problems are interrelated and could be managed more efficiently and effectively with community culture based programs. For example, in attempting to reduce high-school dropout rates, it becomes quickly evident that poverty, obesity, poor dietary habits, low self-esteem, unsafe driving, poor school performance, non-participation in sports, unintended pregnancy, substance abuse, drug commerce, and failure to complete high school are highly interrelated and possibly part of the same syndrome. Categorical programs also have the potential to divide community residents according to their allegiance to specific diseases or health problems. Pediatricians, parents, and teachers, for instance, will claim that services for children should be the highest priority because they represent the future of the community. Cardiologists and their patients and families, on the other hand, will argue that cardiovascular disease is a leading cause of death and should be given priority funding. And geriatricians and families will cite the cost benefits of managing the care of older citizens at home to advocate for the prioritization of that population.

CULTURE BASED PLANNING

Given the history and magnitude of state, regional, and national health planning, why have efforts to control cost ended up costing more and producing less? Why do identified solutions fail to produce the desired outcomes of longer, healthy lives and the elimination of health disparities? And why do health disparities exist in a country so rich in resources? At least some of the answers to such questions lie, once again, in the disinclination to take into account that murky, complex, socio-economic matrix that makes up a community's culture. The disappointments of both resource-based and population-based plans are not because they were focused on resources or population health, but rather because they were *not* focused on local context, values, beliefs, behavior, and social organization.

When city health planners decided to close a small, underutilized, formerly religion-affiliated hospital providing limited services, they thought community residents would be better served by a nearby medical center and that resources derived from the closure would be applied to designated initiatives that would improve the health of the community. What the planners did not count on was strong community opposition to the closure of a hospital with a century-long history of serving local residents—as a health facility and as an employer. As such, the hospital in question gleaned both sentiment and support from community residents. The dominant ethnic/religious group in the community perceived this action as yet another threat and disrespect for its traditions. Champions for retaining the hospital included community members, labor unions, hospital employees, and powerful politicians working on behalf of their constituencies. To the citizens of this community, the closing of the hospital was not just about rational health care. In fact, it really was not about health care at all. It was about religion, politics, economics, and the social representation of community life. It was about community self-determination.

As this case demonstrates, health planning is likely to generate community opposition when the stakeholders have not been part of the process, and when the cultural matrix of both the problem and solution has not been considered. Although popular sentiment and modest employment opportunities cannot and should not sustain a costly and ineffective facility, a culturally informed plan could have included converting the hospital to another kind of health facility that would retain employees. It could have enlisted the community stakeholders—for example, hospital workers, political leaders, and religious leaders—early in the planning, and perhaps have arranged a neighborhood event that celebrated the hospital and its contribution to the community.

A culturally informed plan is one that makes sense to the people who live in the community (Young Laing, 2009). Plans for preventing and treating alcohol abuse in a community where the consumption of alcohol has both social and economic value will be different from one designed for a community in which the consumption of alcohol is regarded as deviant behavior. Plans to reduce the rate of adolescent pregnancy will be different in a town where the high-school graduation–college–marriage–pregnancy sequence is embedded in the culture as opposed to one in which pregnancy at a young age is regarded as a normal and welcome event, signaling transition to womanhood. Likewise, programs for reducing the consumption of high-cholesterol foods may not be welcome in communities where dairy and beef production is the economic base.

Adolescent obesity constitutes a serious and enduring national problem. Identified as a national goal in *Healthy People 2000, 2010, and 2020,* a reduction in the proportion of adolescents who are overweight or obese has been a leading health indicator. Yet, after more than two decades, there has been virtually no progress made. In addition, as the following statistics indicate, the racial and ethnic disparities in teenage obesity have not only persisted, but widened (Ogden and Carroll, 2010).

Between 1988 and 1994, and 2007 and 2008, the prevalence of obesity in girls increased as follows (Healthy People 2020):

- From 8.9% to 14.5% among non-Hispanic white girls

- From 16.3% to 29.2% among non-Hispanic black girls

- From 13.4% to 17.4% among Mexican-American girls

The prevalence of obesity in boys also increased:

- From 11.6% to 16.7% among non-Hispanic white boys

- From 10.7% to 19.8% among non-Hispanic black boys

- From 14.1% to 26.8% among Mexican-American boys

Using this example to compare planning approaches, resource-based planning would address the burgeoning problem of adolescent obesity in our society by increasing products and services for those seeking treatment. These might include the following:

- Weight-loss clinics with an emphasis on teenagers

- Weight-loss pharmaceutical products marketed to youth

- Special education for providers who work with teenagers

- Gastric bypass and bariatric surgery

- Self-help groups, books, and programs on weight management that would appeal to teenagers

Population-based planning would identify at-risk groups (African-American girls, for example) and try to reduce risk to this population through prevention. These efforts might include the following:

- High-school–based nutrition-education programs

- Regulations requiring the labeling of caloric, carbohydrate, and fat content on foods typically consumed by adolescents

- Working with fast-food restaurants to offer healthy alternatives

- High-school exercise and fitness programs for non-athletes

- Cooking classes for teens

Interestingly, none of these solutions has been effective in stemming the rates of obesity in the 12- to 19-year-old population.

As with countless other national health problems for which medical treatment and/or lifestyle changes are required (for example, smoking, alcohol and drug consumption, unprotected sex, lack of exercise), the determinants and the solutions are most likely found in the cultural context of the communities in which they occur. How, for example, are dietary practices and food consumption related to local school menus, vending machines, recreation, housing, communication, ethnic traditions and celebrations, the economy, and the beliefs and values about food that guide eating behavior? Which community institutions would be most effective in addressing obesity (for example, schools, workplaces, places of worship, or health facilities)? How is food consumption linked to school performance, home responsibilities, friendships, and recreation? Basically, when, where, with whom, and why do these teenagers consume food, and what do they eat? It is at the community level that clinical, social, educational, economic, and environmental factors come together to explain and address the multiple factors influencing diet, nutrition, and, ultimately, health.

Culture based planning uses strategies from both resource-based and population-based planning, but expands the epidemiological and problem-based orientation to include cultural inquiry and analysis of the local community. An understanding of local culture enables us to see how problems and solutions are linked to other problems and solutions, and to begin to identify where points of intervention occur. Although overweight and obese adolescence is a national health problem, solutions and policies generated at the suprastructure may not have a predictable outcome at the local infrastructure. Well-intended federal and state programs can sink or swim at the local level, where citizens feel influence and exercise power, where resistance or support is most keenly experienced, and where the complex relationship between people, their environment, and social organizations is most reactive. Those who have been involved in comprehensive health planning for some time can point to national programs for nutrition education, family planning, chemical dependency, prevention, or sanitation that were either redirected or dismantled at the community level, never fulfilling their original intent.

Suggested Activity

Choose a current health problem in your community and outline a resource-based, population-based, and culture based plan.

- What is the health issue or problem? Describe your community.

- What is the resource-based plan? Describe the health care resources that will be required to manage this problem.

- What is the population-based plan? Describe the at-risk populations and the prevention and health promotion strategies you would use.

- What is the culture based plan? Describe the health issue or problem within the context of community life and the culture specific strategies you would use to address it.

CREATING A CULTURALLY INFORMED HEALTHY COMMUNITY AGENDA

In clinical practice, familiar care plans outline the pathways to desired clinical outcomes. Through anticipatory guidance, we also help individuals and families plan for the future so they will have the resilience and flexibility to manage changes in health and development (for example, bringing home a new baby or preparing for retirement as well as managing a chronic illness or preparing a family for a divorce). But planning is so intrinsic to community practice that it is often difficult to separate it as a distinguishable phase or activity. In community practice, creating and sustaining a healthy community infrastructure cannot be accomplished without deliberate, continuous, and long range planning. Combining accountability for the health of whole communities with personal knowledge of and relationships with residents and organizations, the nursing profession has an unparalleled opportunity to activate its long standing vision of promoting healthy communities through long range planning.

Components of the process necessary to create a healthy community infrastructure identified in Healthy People 2020 are outlined here. Once again, while these are presented in sequential format, in reality, these components are linked in a dynamic, continuous, and mutually reinforcing process.

- **Overarching goals:** What are the ultimate purposes of our work?

- **Mission, vision, and values:** What are we going to do? Why are we doing this? What are the principles that guide our work?

- **Stakeholders:** What is the existing health planning structure and organization? How is it linked to other planning organizations? Who are the community individuals currently involved in planning, and which individuals and groups are not at the planning table?

- **Objectives:** What accomplishments will we use to indicate our progress toward a healthy community? What criteria will we use to select objectives? What criteria will we use to prioritize our objectives? How will we measure our objectives?

■ **Strategies:** How will we implement our objectives? What is our plan of work? What is our activity plan? What is our strategic plan?

OVERARCHING GOALS

Creating a healthy community is not unlike creating a healthy nation. In Healthy People 2020, more than 600 objectives were identified as part of a national agenda for health improvement. Although many of the focus areas and objectives from 2010 were continued in Healthy People 2020, 13 new objectives were added to reflect contemporary health and social concerns. Similarly, the myriad objectives included in a healthy community agenda will shift and adjust to accommodate the inevitable changes that take place within the community, the wider society, and the world.

Overarching goals, in contrast, are broader, more enduring, and serve as a framework within which objectives and strategies are selected and implemented. Building community capacity to meet the overarching goals of Healthy People 2020 requires the engagement of all citizens and groups in ownership of the community's health and welfare, resulting in an empowered community infrastructure that is equipped to manage the relationship between environment and population, now and in the future. As culture workers and capacity builders, we are accountable for bringing agencies, groups, and organizations together to design a healthy future for the community.

VISION, MISSION, AND VALUES

An important strength of the Healthy People series is that each one begins with a vision statement that guides community health planning and anchors the process with a common purpose. For Healthy People 2020, it is simply, "A society in which all people live long, healthy lives." This statement has the power to bring varied and often disparate groups to a common goal. Although there may be disagreement about the strategies and activities comprising a healthy community agenda, each one ultimately must contribute to the vision.

The vision states what or who you are and why you are engaged in this process—usually, the simpler the vision, the better. A mission statement, on the other hand, describes what you are here to do and often what distinguishes you from others with a similar mission. The mission of a college of nursing may be to prepare the next generation of leaders in the profession. The mission of a hospital may be to provide patient-centered acute care. The mission of a restaurant may be to serve fresh and wholesome food to discerning customers. Usually, mission statements are longer than vision statements and are more explicit. For example, the mission statement for Healthy People 2020 is to strive to do the following:

- Identify nationwide health improvement priorities.

- Increase public awareness and understanding of the determinants of health, disease, and disability, and the opportunities for progress.

- Provide measurable objectives and goals that are applicable at the national, state, and local levels.

- Engage multiple sectors to take action to strengthen policies and improve practices that are driven by the best available evidence and knowledge.

- Identify critical research, evaluation, and data-collection needs.

Value statements identify the principles by which a mission is accomplished. An example of a value statement is, "all people have the right to health and health care." This statement lets everyone know that this value cannot be violated in the pursuit of the mission. It is not an empirical statement, but rather an ethical/philosophical statement grounded in societal and professional norms. Although it is important to clarify and endorse values to guide the planning process, ultimately, it is in actual behavior that the true values or norms of a society are exposed. The realities of widespread health disparities and disenfranchisement of whole sectors of community residents probably reveal the most about our social values regarding who is entitled to health and who is not. An objective appraisal of our highly entrepreneurial health care system might indicate that the true driving value of contemporary health care is that sophisticated and expensive medical procedures will be reserved only for those who have the ability to pay; however, such a statement would be inconsistent with the normative values endorsed by our society. During the planning process, it is useful to acknowledge the range of values that are likely to be expressed and to identify some shared value as a starting point. Although Healthy People 2020 does not have a specific value statement, its guiding values are evident in the vision, mission, and overarching goals: health equity, good science, high quality, equal access, public awareness, prevention, community engagement, and interdisciplinary partnerships.

Suggested Activity

Do the following:

- Write a vision statement for your community project.
- Write a mission statement for your community project
- List the values that guide your project.

STAKEHOLDERS AND COMMUNITY ENGAGEMENT

In most localities, both public and private health care organizations (for example, health departments, community alliances, strategic-planning groups, and associations of care providers) already are deeply involved in health planning. Using community inquiry data, the first step is to identify the organizations and individuals currently engaged in planning for the health of a community. As described in Chapter 4, "Discovering the Culture of Your Community," and Chapter 5, "Determining the Health of Your Community," the characteristics of the planning infrastructure and its membership will vary with the community, reflecting local values and social organization. Preferably, the health planning infrastructure will articulate with other community organizations and planning groups (for example, education, arts and culture, religious organizations, economic development, housing, transportation) and with other health planning organizations in neighboring communities or at the municipal, county, state, and national levels. This coordination will help to ensure the most cost-effective and -coordinated planning.

Citizen participation is not new in health planning. From the Hill-Burton Act in 1946 to the mandated citizen majority in the 1974 Health Planning Act, community partnerships have been a hallmark of public health practice. Although the early years of mandated citizen involvement led to some disillusionment regarding the role and function of citizens (Steckler and Herzog, 1979), contemporary provider groups and organizations usually welcome the presence of community residents who not only will interpret the community and its culture for others, but will facilitate the implementation of health plans. As we know, however, a community citizenry is not necessarily of one mind. Although planning goals come from an assessment of community needs, they are modified and prioritized *vis-à-vis* the availability of resources and competing community interests. It is therefore normal in the planning process for goal-setting to be sometimes contentious and politicized as various groups within the community compete for limited resources. It also is normal for citizen representatives to be as self-interested as any other board member and to disagree with other self-interested citizens, perhaps more than they disagree with the professional members. Finally, although community partnerships are essential for a successful community health practice, they are not a substitute for the systematic assessment and analysis of the community culture.

The very selection of community stakeholders to serve on a board or coalition must be grounded in cultural knowledge about who they are in the community; to whom they are related; their political, religious, and occupational affiliations; their public interests; and potential conflicts of interest.

The health of a community is the shared responsibility of all its residents, families, and organizations. One measure of successful planning is the extent to which it provides the opportunity for the voices of all community members to be heard through active involvement in subcommittees, consultation, or public hearings. Health disparities and quality-of-life issues, in particular, mandate the engagement of multiple sectors of community life, such as education, religion, government, the economy, and recreation. In culture based planning, local stakeholders become invested not only in solving current problems, but in understanding the culture of their community, identifying and prioritizing health needs, and creating a healthy community agenda for the future.

During the 1970s, a community service group from the U.S. was working with villagers on a Caribbean island. They noticed a large, two-story building, housing older and disabled villagers. Because the building had only one staircase, disabled persons living on the second floor were unable to access the outdoors. To address this problem, the U.S group—in partnership with officials from key island organizations—planned and built a wheelchair-accessible ramp from the second floor to the yard surrounding the building. While this intervention was intended to enhance the lives of the confined residents, it permitted confused, disabled persons to go down the ramp alone and become lost in the surrounding rainforest and even drown at sea. While the intent to provide access to the outdoors was a good and culturally appropriate effort, with only two caregivers to assist more than 50 older and disabled residents, the results were disastrous. A systematic culturally informed community health assessment and a consultation with local residents and the caregivers might have predicted and prevented the sad outcomes of this well-intended plan.

OBJECTIVES

Objectives refer to the specific measurable or documented targets used to trace the progress necessary to reach goals.

Identifying Objectives

Our community health assessment from Chapter 5 revealed the explicit objectives we want to include in our healthy community agenda. As described in the Community Tool Box (http://ctb.ku.edu), the objectives identified in Healthy People 2020 tell us how we are doing in achieving the nationwide agenda for health. They are specific and calculable milestones to be accomplished at a certain level and within a certain timeframe. To be included in Healthy People 2020, objectives must:

■ Be prevention-oriented.

■ Drive action that will work toward the achievement of the proposed targets.

■ Be useful and reflect issues of national importance.

- Be measurable and address a range of issues.

- Be continuous and comparable.

- Be supported by the best available scientific evidence.

- Address population disparities.

- Be valid, reliable, and drawn from nationally representative data.

No single Healthy People 2020 objective will apply to all communities; nor will all objectives apply to any one community. Similarly, a healthy community agenda is composed of many objectives, some of which will apply only to certain sectors of the community, but in concert, will improve the health of the whole community. Although it is likely that many community objectives will be similar to those in Healthy People 2020 (with its 42 broadly applicable topic areas), and may use the same measures for progress, the identification of both objectives and strategies begins with the community. The objective to improve public high-school completion rates, for example, may apply to many communities, but the causes of the problem and the strategies for the solution will vary significantly from community to community.

One of the objectives of Healthy People 2010 was to eliminate ethnic disparities in high-school completion rates. Dropping out of school is associated with deferred employment, poverty, and poor health. The target of 90% set for this objective was consistent with the national education goals to increase the high-school graduation rate of all ethnic groups to at least 90%. In 1996, only 62% of Hispanic/Latino and 83% of African-American youth, aged 18 to 24, had completed high school, compared to 92% for white, non-Hispanic youth (Healthy People 2010).

In Healthy People 2020, the health and social problems of teenagers and their impact on the neighborhoods where they live were considered sufficiently important to create a new topic area for adolescent health with 11 objectives and 24 measures. The 2010 high-school completion rate objective, which was not achieved, was modified in 2020 to "Increase the proportion of students who graduate with a regular diploma four years after starting ninth grade." A target of 82.4% was established, using a baseline of a 74.9% average graduation rate for public school students graduating with a regular diploma in 2007–08. Because the high-school dropout rate for non-Hispanic white adolescents was 92%, using an overall dropout rate will still capture ethnic differences.

In one community, low high-school completion rates may reflect the need for teenagers to economically assist their families by entering the workforce while still in high school. In another community, high-school completion may be linked to a high rate of teenage pregnancy. In still another, it may be associated with drug use and commerce. If residents remain unconvinced of the importance of a problem, its solution will require a different strategy than if there were widespread community support. For example, in some communities, it may be inappropriate to focus on reducing the rate of adolescent pregnancy to achieve the goal of 82.4% high-school completion rates. The optimal life stage in which to become pregnant is guided by cultural tradition, religious canons, and socioeconomic factors. In communities that are more comfortable with teen pregnancy, a more effective solution for improving high-school completion rates may focus on removing the barriers that prevent teen mothers from completing high school rather than not becoming pregnant in the first place.

Prioritizing Objectives

A culturally integrated approach, using the community's timeframe, will create an effective and realistic schedule for pursuing a healthy community agenda. The overarching goals of the healthy community agenda provide a useful set of criteria by which to prioritize objectives (Healthy People 2020):

- What is the extent of risk to the entire community if the problem is unresolved?

- Is there a need to resolve one problem before another problem can be addressed?

- To what extent will the solution of one problem solve many other problems?

Our cultural knowledge of the community assists us to forecast more accurately in the determination of the relative importance and timing of initiatives. Forecasting is the process of predicting what would happen if one objective were selected to precede another, as well as what would happen if nothing were done about the problem. For example, given the close relationship between education and personal health behavior, mental health, family dysfunction, crime, employment, substance abuse, and domestic violence, an extraordinarily compelling case can be made for increasing the rates of high-school completion.

Finally, the reconciliation of professionally identified needs and community identified demands is an important part of priority-setting. Residents may feel, for example, that adolescent sexuality is a serious problem that must be addressed in the context of high-school completion. In contrast, the provider community may be less concerned with the relatively few occurrences of adolescent pregnancy compared with documented, widespread cigarette smoking by adolescents. The goal is to bring the community perspective and the provider perspective together in a culturally informed, prioritized plan for adolescent health.

Measuring Objectives

An effective healthy community agenda requires not only prioritized objectives, but also indicators that you have achieved them. Once the objectives have been prioritized, they must be translated into measurable outcomes, or targets, that will demonstrate the attainment of a goal. The objective to improve public high-school completion rates is both data-driven (from an analysis of education statistics) and value-driven (from the principles of social justice and equity). It must be stated, however, in a way that would make progress measurable. What specific behaviors or events are desired? The objective would then be phrased in behavioral or measurable terms. Such as, the target rate set for timely high-school completion in Healthy People 2020 is 82.4%.

In addition to stating the target outcome, it is necessary to state the timeframe within which the outcome is expected. This will depend on the nature and extent of the problem, the resources available, and the culture of the community. In some communities, it may be realistic to say improvement in public high-school completion rates could be 95% in four years, while others may require a longer period to get to 80%. Using interim benchmarks to revisit outcomes on an annual basis, the timeframe also should be consistent with the length of time necessary to measure the effects. Increasing the rate of high-school completion, for example, may take much longer than improving teenage driving safety, which is more amenable to regulation and policy. Successful accomplishment of interim benchmarks or short term goals is helpful in providing encouragement to planners and stakeholders. It is important, however, that long term, truly consequential goals representing real progress in improving health and reducing disparities not be forgotten in the wake of short term success.

STRATEGIES

Strategies describe how we are going to accomplish the objectives we've selected to achieve our overarching goals. The first step is to review the literature to see what others have done in similar situations. These best practices and/or evidence-based intervention programs are then evaluated in the context of our particular community for cultural appropriateness and feasibility. Some may not work at all; others may simply need to be strategically modified for cultural congruence. Good strategies will be consistent with the vision and mission of the plan, within the context of the community. If the mission is to create a healthier community, how does the strategy of having more educated citizens contribute to that mission? Effective strategies also will acknowledge the culture and complexity of communities and build on their cultural capital. Depending on the objective and on the cultural context, the strategies and interventions will vary greatly from those that apply to relatively few sectors of the community. For example, lead screening in a particular neighborhood with older housing will involve different interventions from those that involve the whole community such as disaster preparedness or transforming all vacant city lots into urban gardens.

Healthy People 2020 identified five separate kinds of strategies, although most plans end up being combinations of these five. For example, the five types of strategies to increase the rates of high-school completion include the following:

- Education, information, and skill enhancement (for example, offering continuing education for teachers to identify signs of sexual abuse in adolescents)

- Services and support (for example, offering psychological first-aid programs to adolescents) (Everly & Flynn, 2006)

- Reducing barriers and increasing opportunities (for example, offering an alternative high-school completion program for adolescents who have to work to help support their families)

- Modifying the outcome of efforts (for example, creating incentives such as lower car insurance rates for teens who remain in school and have at least a B average)

- Creating policies (for example, permitting pregnant adolescents to remain in their high schools)

Two communities can manifest the same problem but will mandate different solutions because of differences in cultural context. Determining the best strategies is accomplished through a descriptive and comparative analysis of the problem in relation to the context of community life. By mapping, describing, and charting cultural information about our teenage group in the community in which they live, we determine the cultural capital as well as the barriers that will need to be addressed. Identifying interventions for improving the rate of high-school completion, for example, requires comparing the lives of at-risk teenagers with the larger populations of teenagers in relation to community culture (that is, the physical environment, the characteristics of the population, and the social organization and relationships that link individuals and groups to each other and to the environment).

PUBLIC HIGH-SCHOOL COMPLETION: CONTEXTUAL ANALYSIS

Objective: Improve high-school completion rates	Population: adolescents	Target population: adolescents at risk
Physical environment: space and time	Where do adolescents live (which neighborhoods)? Where do teenagers spend their time? How do teenagers organize their day? Where do they recreate?	Where do target teens live (which neighborhoods)? Where do target teens spend their time? How do target teens spend their day Where do they recreate?
The population	How many adolescents are in the community? What are the demographics? Sex Religion Ethnicity Class Residence Grammar school Housing Economics	How many at-risk adolescents are in the community? What are the demographics? Sex Religion Ethnicity Class Residence Grammar school Housing Economics
Social Organization	What are community organizations for adolescents? What are the value and belief systems of adolescents? How do adolescents organize and relate to community organizations? Economic Political Domestic Religious Education Recreation Voluntary How are adolescents horizontally stratified and vertically segmented?	What are community organizations for at-risk adolescents? What are the value and belief systems of at-risk adolescents? How do at-risk adolescents organize and relate to community organizations? Economic Political Domestic Religious Education Recreation Voluntary How are at-risk adolescents horizontally stratified and vertically segmented?

From this cultural information about our target group in the community context, we begin to determine how various local institutions, individuals, and groups can be identified to address the problem. If young people have to leave school to help support their families, the strategies for improving high-school completion rates will be very different from strategies used in a community in which a high drop-out rate is attributed to the use and sale of illicit drugs. Depending on the context of the problem, there will be different cultural capital, different stakeholders, different timeframes, and different strategies. Successful community advocacy and partnership are related directly to (1) how well community cultural information is collected, organized, and applied and (2) the effectiveness of the relationships established with community residents and groups.

BUILDING A CONSTITUENCY FOR CULTURE BASED ACTION: DO WE NEED IT? WHO SHOULD BE ON IT?

Traditionally, nurses have derived their influence from their ministrations. The counsel, care, and comfort they provide to patients and their families—both continuously and in times of crisis—are powerful means for establishing and securing relationships. To build a community wide base of support, however, our authority must reach beyond the private domain of home and family and into the public arena. Community constituencies are built by both knowing and being known by the key citizens and organizations in all their various dimensions. Issues of health and illness potentially affect every member of a community, either directly or indirectly, and community health nurses are experts on how people can stay well and manage health problems. That expertise has a powerful influence on community residents. As prominent members of the community whose mission is highly valued, public health nurses have access to influential members of their communities. Unfortunately, most nurses are unaware of the magnitude of their influence and use it infrequently, even though the amount and nature of their contact with all sectors of the population would be the envy of any legislator. Politicians, on the other hand, are acutely aware of the influence nurses command, both as individuals and as a profession that has generated the admiration, respect, and confidence of community residents. Legislators and other public officials are eager to make the acquaintance of the nurses and to work with them on a variety of health and social issues.

Identifying and making personal contact with influential residents is essential for building community relations, and probably *the* fundamental skill of successful public health practice. Even in the early stages of community assessment, it is possible to recognize potential constituents and get some idea of what you can provide that is important to them. This might include suggesting to a young television reporter that she will be first on your list of people to call with an interesting story about the health of the community, or letting a political official know that your office would be happy to provide her health aide with the necessary statistics to use in her next speech. Or it could be as simple as a personal connection—for example, graduating from the same college, playing bridge, or sharing Swedish ancestry. One of the best ways to meet an influential person is to be introduced by another influential person; before any meeting is over, it's important to ask whether there is anyone else in the community that your influential contact thinks you should meet. Additionally, it is important to remember that your role in the community renders you an influential person who will be called upon for your expertise. The various roles and multiple positions that community persons such as school principals, bank presidents, nurses, pastors, or Rotary officers hold in the community—and how they are linked to one another—are key factors as community nurses go about establishing new relationships.

Finally, one of the most important vehicles for connecting community practitioners with influential decision-makers used to engage the influential members of a community is a community advisory board. The choice of whom to invite to serve on an advisory board should derive directly from the roles and positions of these individuals in relation to the community culture and their capacity to assist in building a power base for a healthy community. The real value of such boards is not widespread citizen participation or even representation. Those goals can be achieved in a number of other ways. Rather, community advisory boards should extend the influence of community health nurses. Members typically are drawn from the local power structure and are likely to sit on other community boards as well. Of course, it is incumbent on public health nurses to give back by volunteering to serve on advisory boards in the many diverse sectors of the community—the city finance committee, an urban-planning task force, or the board of education.

Suggested Activity

Do the following:

- From your community assessment, list six individuals or groups who should be members of your community constituency, your rationale for choosing each person, and what strategies will you use to recruit them.

Who	Why	How

Recruiting and engaging stakeholders in formulating goals, objectives, and strategies lays the groundwork for a citizen action that is culturally informed and community specific. Grounded in the overarching goals of Healthy People 2020, planning in partnership is essential for creating a better future.

LEADING CULTURALLY INFORMED COMMUNITY ACTION

Making the broad, far-reaching changes that will achieve health equity, eliminate disparities, create healthy environments, and promote quality of life for all requires bringing stakeholders together for system level action. This chapter takes us through the complex process of leading change by putting a culturally informed healthy community agenda into action.

CHAPTER 7 OBJECTIVES

- Distinguish between the conflict and consensus models of public health action and use them appropriately.

- Identify the special challenges of communities as clients.

- Apply the principles for building effective coalitions.

- Distinguish between primary and secondary target groups in mobilizing community action.

- Distinguish between a conservative and culturally preservative action plan.

- Understand the principles of a culturally informed public health case statement.

BUILDING CAPACITY THROUGH CITIZEN ENGAGEMENT

Building capacity for community action and change is not just about creating partnerships with community residents and groups to solve specific health problems. Rather, it is a perpetual set of activities that begins with assembling and maintaining an inventory of the community's cultural capital and continues with engaging individuals and organizations in building community capacity (McKay and Hewlett, 2009). Just as clinicians are responsible for collecting, applying, and communicating comprehensive knowledge about their patients, community health practitioners are the custodians of knowledge about the community. We are accountable for ensuring that cultural information is collected, organized, and then employed to enhance the public's health. Creating a sustainable, healthy community equipped to accommodate both challenges and opportunities and to manage problems as they occur requires culturally informed leadership.

GUIDING CHANGE: A CULTURALLY PRESERVATIVE APPROACH

Change cannot be considered out of context. The nature, extent, and speed of planned change depend on the problems being addressed and the cultural milieu in which they occur. The mandate in public health practice is not change for the sake of change, but rather change for the purpose of ensuring and promoting the health of the public. This may or may not require major alterations in community life, and before planners determine how change should be accomplished, they must first determine whether change is necessary. The goal of culture based planning is not to accelerate change, nor to restrain it, but rather to manage it with minimal upheaval and cost while providing significant benefit to the community. A major challenge for contemporary communities is to generate a community health plan that has sufficient flexibility as well as durability to survive in a rapidly changing society.

Effective capacity building is grounded in an understanding and appreciation of local traditions. This culturally preservative approach to civic action is not to be confused with an incremental or conservative approach. The preservative approach is based on the notion that it is possible to accomplish profound and often very rapid change with minimal disruption by casting change in the context of community culture. The effectiveness of health action is related directly to our familiarity with the logic of local customs and behavior and how community life is organized. On first entering a community, our attention typically is drawn to its problems and limitations. As we come to know the culture of our community client better, however, many of the features of community life that appear, at first, to be weaknesses may, in fact, turn out to be its strengths. Behavior that seems almost self-defeating becomes perfectly understandable when viewed within the cultural framework of community life.

> To promote quality of life for rural elders, the county nurse arranged to pick up their medications twice a week at a less-expensive national chain pharmacy located in a city where she resided. To her surprise, the elders preferred to continue purchasing their medications at their local pharmacy, where they paid significantly more. At first, this behavior appeared to be irrational. A cultural inquiry of the community, however, revealed many features about this rural community that were not immediately obvious. The pharmacy was a family-owned business that had served the community for generations. The current pharmacist and her husband lived in the neighborhood and attended the same church as many of their customers. Their children attended the local public school, where the husband taught fifth grade. The pharmacy sponsored many community events and organizations, including a Little League baseball team and a winning high-school girls' basketball team. Without the advantages of a volume business, the pharmacy charged residents more than they would pay through a national pharmacy chain. Yet to not patronize this local business would have offended a well-known family and constituted a serious breach of community culture.

Community residents understand these subtleties and can talk about the value of having a pharmacist who knows you, who is willing to get up in the middle of the night when someone needs medication right away, and who will give you a month or two to pay, if necessary. The residents of this community have a relationship with their pharmacist. They are committed to her, and she to them. Disregarding the patterns and institutions that have been established over decades would seriously jeopardize the building of relationships for community collaboration. Rather than focusing exclusively on the shortcomings of community life or attempting to organize what already is organized, successful community action must begin with respect for local values and traditions. We must be willing to suspend our judgment until we build the relationships with residents that permit us to discover the internal logic of our community client.

MODELS FOR ACTION

Trying to get things done to enhance the current and future health of communities can be a very complicated process. We often are challenged by unanticipated conflict and controversy in working with communities we assumed to be unified in purpose but, in fact, are composed of individuals and groups with divergent preferences and priorities. We have known for over half a century that opposing community factions can be found in even the tiniest villages (Wellin, 1955), but it was not until the introduction of ethnography into public health science that the realities of communities as unwieldy, complicated, and heterogeneous matrices were revealed (Bibeau, 1997; Drevdahl, 2002). Nevertheless, the definition of communities as composed of like-minded citizens united by a common purpose for collective action has continued to permeate public health theory and practice (Bibeau, 1997; Clark, 2007; Davis, 2000; Minkler, 2005; Rosen, 1954; Rothman, 2008).

These different perceptions reflect fundamentally different theories about the nature of communities. One is that communities are held together by a common ideology and value system. The other is that communities are held together by the diversity of values and goals and the capacity of members to meet each other's needs. Applying these two paradigms to the familiar example of a college or university, we might say that students, faculty, and administrators are held together by a shared reverence for the generation and transfer of knowledge. But another way to look at it would be to say that students, faculty, and administrators all have quite different goals, values, and reasons for being there and are held together through a complex exchange of knowledge, money, and services. Like all communities, some things are shared by all the members of the university community, such as pride in a winning basketball team, while others are not, such as the need to increase the cost of tuition.

In community health practice, these two theories about what holds communities together have generated two different models for leading change:

- **The consensus model:** The long standing consensus model assumes communities are defined by a shared set of core values around which members can be organized to reach agreement and achieve common goals (Minkler, 2005). Change is centered on achieving community wide collaboration, including endorsement by the existing power structure. The methods typically used in the consensus model are enhancing communication, moral and rational persuasion, and building rapport. This definition has underpinned community health action and promoted strategies for change such as values clarification, public education, exchange of ideas, and opportunities for relationship-building and communication.

- **The conflict model:** The conflict model, proposed by the founder of modern community organizing, Saul Alinsky (1971), assumes the existence of inherent conflicts and competition in all human groups, including communities. It is based on the belief that self-interest, as well as the common good, guide the behavior of most people. Rather than stressing the commonalities among community members, the conflict model takes into account status differences, rival affiliations, and power relationships. In the conflict model, sweeping change in a community is likely to require realignment of power rather than working with the existing power structure. Acknowledging vested interests, multiple community roles, conflicting values, and power struggles, the existing decision-making process is altered through social affiliations and political action. In a factory, for example, management needs the human labor provided by workers, and workers need the income provided by management. In this exchange, both parties give something and get something. Change, therefore, can take place by one of the parties withholding what the other wants.

The conflict model does not always involve resistance. It often means building bridges between groups that normally have little contact with one another so that members can get to know each other as human beings. When this happens, stereotypes are likely to break down and people begin to bring their reference groups together in a spirit of cooperation. Once again, these bridges are not predicated necessarily on shared values, good will, or humanitarian interests, but rather on the notion that each group has something the other needs or wants. By understanding the nature of self-interest, relationships can be facilitated between and among people who can accomplish their own goals while promoting the health of the public. In other words, the way to deal with vested interests is to understand them and apply them. Rather than be put off by what may be construed as avarice and opportunism, self-interest can be the pillar for formulating a strategy that will accomplish a healthy community agenda.

> In an Eastern city, parents requested that the city council designate certain blocks as "play" streets so they could open fire hydrants on hot summer days. Some councilors endorsed this endeavor because they believed the safety and quality of life for children was important. Others had little interest in the project but supported it because their fellow councilors had supported their causes in the past. Together, their backing resulted in a sufficiently broad base of community support to counter opposition from residents who felt inconvenienced by the closing of streets.

At first, the conflict model may appear to be Machiavellian and manipulative, but the fact that people differ in their commitment to what we may define as a worthy cause is simply a reflection of different priorities. Some citizens will support programs for elders but be indifferent to the disabled; others will support adolescent programs but disregard the homeless. In the conflict model, whether people give money to support a community health initiative because they believe the project is wholesome or morally right or because they earn a tax deduction is immaterial. Similarly, it does not matter whether a politician supports a public health policy change because it will improve the health of the public or because it will win votes. What matters is that we have been effective in building relationships to mobilize support for a healthy community agenda. Finally, it is important to remember that what is "right" in community life is seldom black or white. Practically all people live in a world of shifting priorities and contradictions and claim a morality that they cannot possibly practice to its fullest. Most people, for example, endorse both freedom of the press and the protection of individual privacy. If a highly regarded person is the subject of an unflattering front-page story, community residents may find themselves supporting the right to privacy. On the other hand, the same residents may invoke freedom of the press to publicly discredit a less highly regarded individual.

Advocates of the consensus model cite its unifying capacity, bringing various groups together to work for a common purpose, overcoming resistance to change and developing a sense of pride in being part of something that is bigger than one's self or even one's family. Advocates of the conflict model contend that change achieved through consensus is comparatively trivial and will have little impact on the social and economic dislocations that are at the root of poor health and health disparities. According to the conflict model, the reason people don't want to change is not because humans have an inherent resistance to change, but because they have a vested interest in the status quo. Whether change is described as disorganizing or reorganizing depends on where one stands in the shifting control of resources. Both the consensus and conflict strategies have a place in empowering groups to action, but when and how they are used should be grounded in the cultural information derived from the culturally informed community health assessment. According to Bibeau (1997), the lack of success in health promotion and prevention in North America and throughout the world can be attributed to the failure to acknowledge the complexities of community culture and the reflexive endorsement of action strategies that make assumptions about cultural homogeneity in communities.

THE ROLE OF THE NURSE IN COMMUNITY ACTION

In clinical practice, nurses understand the significance of establishing relationships with their patients to increase the effectiveness of their interventions. Organizing whole communities for civic action, however, offers a different set of challenges that reflect the complexity and diversity of community clients. Nurses are accustomed, for example, to establishing a sense of confidence and trust with patients and their families as they become active and essential participants in their plans of care. In community health, it is equally imperative to establish a strong and trusting relationship with clients and engage them in community action. But because communities are composed of competing populations, groups, and institutions, establishing a trusting relationship with one segment of the community could generate concern in another segment. Even the appearance of an exclusive affiliation with one community group could compromise one's effectiveness in working with the community as a whole. A community nurse who routinely attends a Methodist church, for example, may need to demonstrate his or her respect for other religions in the town or neighborhood by meeting with their leaders and denominations.

Community practitioners become, in effect, ex-officio members of the community, but they are not just *any* member of the community. They occupy a special role, relative to other residents, that carries both privileges and obligations. On the one hand, they have more personal freedom than other members of the community have and typically are judged by a different set of standards. Nurses are permitted—even expected—to develop relationships with all members of the community, including its outcasts, and to visit areas of the community that would be considered off-limits to some residents. They also are privileged to ask highly personal questions and to explore the more intimate details of people's lives. On the other hand, the nurse's position and special role within the community carries certain constraints and responsibilities. Because nurses are reservoirs of knowledge about the personal aspects of residents, they are not privileged to participate in the casual gossip and speculation afforded to most members of the community without seriously undermining their credibility and the community's confidence.

Building community relations becomes even more complicated when community health nurses reside in the community where they work. As residents, nurses are complex stakeholders, ordinarily occupying several positions or roles that could result in conflicting allegiances. Some public health departments screen employees' ancillary jobs as a requirement of employment because some kinds of work may be perceived to undermine the department's credibility. At the same time, being a resident can augment effectiveness. If community health nurses have children attending local schools, for example, they will have a personal, as well as professional, interest in street safety and school health. If the owner of the local industry is a relative or friend, the nurse may be well-positioned to negotiate for occupational safety improvements. For public health nurses who reside in the communities where they work, community members are not just the target population; they are their children's teachers, their spouse's employer, their rabbi, or their mechanic. For the residents, the public health nurse is not just a nurse, but also a neighbor, customer, or fellow club member. It is not impossible for resident nurses to balance and negotiate community relationships; it simply requires thoughtful consideration of their relationships with the individuals and groups that make up the population of the community.

Whether they are residents or not, the ultimate goal of public health practice is to build community capacity. In some respects, building community capacity is not unlike helping individuals and families acquire the skills to successfully manage the problems, losses, crises, and adjustments that are bound to occur over a lifetime. Unlike patients and families, however, communities are matrices where complex and often competing institutions and populations intersect. Public health nurses must work thoughtfully and skillfully with the full range of community leaders and institutions found in almost all communities.

CREATING AN ACTION PLAN FOR A HEALTHY COMMUNITY AGENDA

Chapter 6, "Laying the Foundation for a Healthy Community Agenda," took us from the overarching goal and vision of a prepared, sustainable community through the development of a culturally informed strategic plan for implementing public health objectives. In this chapter, we apply the findings of our community culture inquiry and health assessment to engage a community specific action plan. An action plan (also called a plan of work or an operational plan) identifies the specific activities and events needed to achieve the overarching goals and objectives of the healthy community agenda. The action plan translates program objectives into a community specific plan of work in a detailed description of the what, who, when, and where of the initiative.

The Mobilize, Assess, Plan, Implement, Track (MAP-IT) framework for community action presented in Healthy People 2020 is a useful guide for moving through the process of leading change. MAP-IT alone, however, will not provide the specific strategies required to build community capacity and mobilize civic action within the cultural context of a particular community. We may understand the meaning and importance of *mobilize*, for example, but how do we mobilize in Eau Claire, WI, as opposed to Baton Rouge, LA, or Willits, CA, or Shelburne Falls, MA, or Chicago's west side? To make MAP-IT come alive with the cultural realities of our specific community, the complexities and nuances of local life must be loaded into each category of the framework.

Designing a culturally informed action plan requires an analysis of the problem in relation to the context of community life:

- What is the nature and extent of the problem?

- How does the target population fit into community life?

- What is the community cultural capital that can be applied to this public health problem?

- At what points do the special needs of the target group intersect with community institutions and populations?

- What are the local barriers that will need to be addressed?

To illustrate, let us explore the process of developing a community specific action plan using one of the 13 new topic areas in Healthy People 2020: older adults.

The baby-boomer population (adults born between 1946 and 1964) is one of the fastest-growing age groups in the nation. Because of the advances in public health and health sciences, people in this age group are living longer, but they also are more likely to be living with at least one chronic illness. It is predicted that by 2030, more than 37 million baby boomers (60%) will be managing more than one chronic illness. Even though most elders want to stay in their homes, chronic illness and injury (mostly falls) limit their capacity to remain independent. Prevention and health promotion programs designed to prevent declines from illness and falls are supported by federal government agencies and are included in the Patient Protection and Affordable Care Act. Less than 20% of older adults, however, engage in physical activity (Healthy People, 2020). Moreover, if they *do* acquire illnesses and disabilities, they may have insufficient support (coordination of care, public transportation, neighborhood safety, home reconfiguration, reliable caregivers, specially educated health professionals, and family and social networks) to continue living independently. This is true even though states that invest in such services show lower rates of growth in long term care expenditures. The potentially soaring health care costs associated with expensive hospitalizations, long term care, and rehabilitative services places an enormous burden on the health care system and on every citizen in the United States. Consequently, the overarching goal for older adults in Healthy People 2020—to "improve the health, function, and quality of life of older adults"—involves several objectives aimed at the following:

- Health promotion (exercise, social engagement)

- Prevention of chronic illness (for example, diabetes, arthritis, congestive heart failure) and injury (specifically falls)

- Community support systems (public transportation, safe housing, providers with the knowledge and skill set to address the needs of older adults)

The health and quality of life of older adults is a nationwide issue, but its expression and extent will vary locally. Although programs offered by federal government agencies provide many resources to address the concern, the most-effective health promotion, prevention, and management solutions will be accomplished in the cultural context of communities where elders live out their lives. A culturally informed action plan that will accomplish the objectives and overarching goals outlined in Healthy People 2020 begins with comparing and contextualizing the community's older-adult population according to the three dimensions of community life:

- The physical environment of time and space

- The characteristics of the population

- The social relationships and interactions within the population and between the population and the environment

There are a number of ways to define the population in question, depending on the community as well as the problem. In the following example, the older-adult population is divided into two subpopulations: from 65 to 80 and over 80. Typically, issues of living at home and the importance of effective support services begin to intensify at age 80.

Suggested Activity

Analyze the identified community health issue or concern in relation to its cultural context.

Building Capacity for Healthy Aging: Culture Context Analysis

Objective: Increase the Percentage of Elders Who Reside Independently in Their Homes	Adults Age 65—79	Adults Age 80 and Above
Physical environment: space and time		
Where do they live (which neighborhoods)?		

Objective: Increase the Percentage of Elders Who Reside Independently in Their Homes	Adults Age 65—79	Adults Age 80 and Above
Where do they spend their day? Week? Year?		
Where and when do they go on a daily and weekly basis?		
Where and when do they get together?		
The population		
Number and percentage of elders in the community?		
What are the demographics?		
Age		
Sex		
Religion		
Ethnicity		
Class		
Residence		
Housing		
Length of time in the community		
The social system		
What is their relationship to community institutions?		
Religion		
Economy/workforce/job		
Recreation/sports		
Health care		
Education		
Domestic/family life		
Communication/transportation		

Objective: Increase the Percentage of Elders Who Reside Independently in Their Homes	Adults Age 65—79	Adults Age 80 and Above
Where do they fit in horizontal stratification of community?		
Where do they fit into community vertical segmentation?		

By plotting the two groups of older adults against the matrix of community culture, we secure a deeper understanding of both the strength and vulnerability of these two older-adult populations and how they relate to the larger community. We then can see how our population of interest intersects with the wider community. We discover the cultural capital—the people, institutions, services, and environmental features—that can be mobilized to create the most cost-effective and culturally preservative action plan.

- **The place:** Where and when can we find our two groups of older adults in the community? Are there specific neighborhoods or apartment complexes in which they are more likely to reside, or are they distributed evenly throughout the community? Where and when do they get congregate (restaurants, faith-based institutions, Rotary or Lions club meetings, recreational activities)? How do they use their time, on a daily, weekly, and seasonal basis? For example, do they visit family every weekend? Do they leave (or return) for the winter months?

- **The people:** How many persons in the community are in one of these two age groups? What is the percentage of older adults in the community? In what kind of housing do older adults live (in their own homes, with younger family members, in retirement communities, in assisted-living centers, in skilled-nursing facilities)? How many live alone? How physically close are their families? What are the socio-demographic characteristics of this population (for example, sex, ethnicity, class, religion, income, education, housing, length of time in the community)?

■ **The social organization:** Where do older adults fit into the socioeconomic stratification of the community? For example, are they equally distributed among the classes or do they, as a group, tend to represent the more-powerful or least-powerful strata of the community's class structure? Do they occupy a special segment of the community (long time residents or newcomer retirees; a distinct ethnic category; a seasonal population)? In what ways do older adults participate in community life? What are the community services they use (grocery stores, hairdressers, public transportation, drug stores, dry cleaners, lawn services, legal services)? What are the forms of recreation in which they engage (television, bridge games, casinos, bingo, movies, operas and symphonies, the library)?

From this cultural information about the role and status of our population of interest, we can begin to understand and address how they promote their own health and maintain their preferred lifestyle, such as living in their homes as long as possible. Who are the persons who have a vested interest in their welfare (for example, family members, religious leaders, neighbors, people who deliver the mail, friends, health insurers, hairdressers, grocers, lawn service, or a local car service)? Is the restaurant where they gather a natural location in which to provide health education and group support? Will grocery stores provide shopping and transportation services? Each community will be very different in terms of the stakeholders involved and the kind of action required. Addressing the issue of residential living for older persons in a community where older adults are in daily physical contact with family members is very different from one in which their families live thousands of miles away. There will be different sets of stakeholders, different interventions, and different timeframes, reflecting the cultural distinctions of each community.

No matter which organizational strategy or combination of strategies is used in public health, it must be grounded in the identification and application of community cultural capital—the values, beliefs, events, organizations, physical structures, and citizens required to build public health capacity. By articulating community health goals with the community's culture and sharing the responsibility for community health with designated community members, we can accomplish an effective and sustainable healthy community agenda. This is true whether the specific issue is senior living, child obesity, domestic violence, toxic waste, or summer-recreation safety.

THE MAP-IT FRAMEWORK: MOBILIZE, ASSESS, PLAN, IMPLEMENT, TRACK

Now we are ready to walk through a culturally informed version of the MAP-IT framework for community action.

MOBILIZE

Mobilizing for public health action is about identifying and building relationships with community stakeholders. Each objective in a healthy community agenda gives rise to two kinds of stakeholders, or target populations, needed to engage and accomplish the action plan. Those who are directly affected by the action plan constitute the primary target—the category of individuals or groups for whom the program is intended (for example, senior citizens, migrant workers, or automobile drivers). The secondary target consists of those persons and organizations that may not be affected by the program directly, but are instrumental in facilitating (or impeding) its success. Legislators, for example, are an important secondary target group in sponsoring regulations that will provide safe housing for older adults. Factory owners may be a critical secondary target group for supporting elder-daycare programs for their employees who are caregivers of their elder parents. Children and schools could be secondary targets in a program for children to dissuade their grandparents from smoking. Secondary targets include community decision-makers whose endorsement is needed to accomplish the proposed plan, as well as those who have a vested interest in the project.

The forum for mobilizing stakeholders for civic action is called a coalition. Unlike constituencies, which provide ongoing support and representation for nurses, a coalition is a group of individuals and organizations that has been convened for the express purpose of accomplishing a specific goal. The identification and selection of a coalition is drawn from our community cultural analysis of the problem or issue in the context of the specific culture. Time, for example, is a critical consideration in identifying which legislator to include in the coalition. The choice of legislator will depend not only on voting histories and campaign promises but also on his or her term of office and proximity to the next election. A popular owner of a restaurant in which elders gather routinely, the president of the Rotary club who may himself or herself be over 65, a contractor who can retrofit homes with safety bars and ramps, and the owner of a local business from which many older adults in the community have retired are all potential coalition members.

Each coalition is composed of a different set of individuals, some of whom may be opponents on some issues but have come together for a cause they now have in common. For example, a Catholic priest and a state government representative may work very well together in advancing the health and well-being of older citizens but be in completely different camps when it comes to contraception and sex education in schools. Coalitions are important not only for mobilizing community members for a particular initiative but also for establishing relationships where none existed previously and for engaging all citizens as stakeholders in building capacity. When individuals and groups that ordinarily are on opposite sides of the table have the opportunity to collaborate on a common cause, they also have the opportunity to develop personal relationships that may soften their disagreement on other issues.

Suggested Activity

Applying information from the community culture analysis, list six individuals and/or groups you would ask to serve on a coalition to address your identified community health issue/problem. Identify the value each member brings as well as the potential difficulty each member may pose.

Coalition Membership	Position in Community and Their Value to the Initiative	Potential Barriers or Problems Their Presence May Create

ASSESS

One of the first responsibilities of the coalition members is to acquire an understanding of the problem, issue, or concern as it is expressed in the community, its determinants, and the resources available to address it. For example:

- How large is the over-65 and over-80 population now?

- What will it be in five, 10, and 20 years?

- What is the percentage of this population in relation to the population of the whole community?

- How does it compare to national, state, and local statistics? (This may be an indicator of the availability of national, state, and local resources.)

- How many and what percent of older adults live at home or reside in assisted-living or long term care facilities?

- What are the number, purpose, and percent of hospital admissions and emergency department visits?

- How many seniors who are admitted to the hospital end up never returning to live independently in their homes?

- How many older adults are at risk for having to leave their homes?

- What type and amount of resources are required to increase the number of older adults who reside in their own homes?

    - Physical reconfiguration of homes for easier access

    - Emergency call capability

    - Electronic communication devices

    - Reliable transportation

    - Personal shoppers

- Visiting services

- Assistance with paying bills and home management

- What are the resources already available in the community to address the issue?

- What programs/interventions have been used in other communities to address the same issue?

The purposes of the assessment are as follows:

- To identify the severity and extent of the issue or problem and its impact on local life

- To identify the resources—or cultural capital—available to address the concern

- To discern the applicability of tested programs in similar communities that have produced desired results

The assessment is necessary for prioritizing the action plan and revealing existing local resources that can be mobilized and directed to address the safety and independence of older citizens. Many resources may already exist within a community, but without a culture inquiry, may not be immediately obvious. Here are a few examples:

- In a hilly New England town, the community health nurse invited a local ski resort to donate its used ski poles so older adults could get outside during the winter.

- In a southern community, senior high-school students prepared a laminated list of important phone numbers in large print for older adults living at home and then helped them to input the numbers into their phones for direct dialing.

- With the assistance of a local farmer who donated space in his barn, a community nurse in a Midwest agricultural community created a storage area for used hospital beds, commodes, crutches, canes, and other medical equipment that could be distributed to community residents who needed them.

■ Nursing students assigned to manage the care of adults over the age of 80 living at home were able to reduce depression rates simply by calling three times a week to ask questions about mobility, medication, and social activity.

Using the local cultural capital of a ski resort, a high-school senior civics class, a retired farmer with a large barn, and a college nursing course in gerontology, these communities were able to offer no-cost or low-cost contributions to the health and independence of older adults.

PLAN

Public health action would be simple if you could count on the whole community seeing the importance and logic of supporting a particular initiative when presented with the evidence, and setting aside personal interests to do so. In reality, however, practically all public health initiatives will be received with varying degrees of enthusiasm—from full support to indifference to frank opposition. The individual steps that make up an action plan will help to determine the specific relationships and activities required to make the community's vision a reality. Sometimes, opposition is the product of a simple lack of understanding of the project's mission and can be corrected easily with action steps focused on communication and education. Other times, opposition comes from competition for limited resources, in which case the action-step response may be a trade-off—for example, "I will support your school lunch program if you support my vision screening for older adults program." Reduced transit fares for persons over 65 may be viewed as increasing the tax liability of other citizens and may require appealing to legislators for support, which usually includes supplying them with data about the costs to taxpayers when older adults are not able to live in their own homes.

Healthy People 2020 offers useful guidelines for writing action steps, including the following:

■ What will happen?

■ Who will do what?

- When will it happen?

- What are the other resources required?

- What are the barriers and sources of resistance, and how will they be overcome?

- Who are the collaborators?

The selection of action steps should come from discussion among the entire coalition. This provides opportunities to generate and debate ideas—not only on action steps and priorities, but also on the suitability of best practices or evidence-based interventions that have been used in other communities. Ample time must be provided for open discussion of the ideas and concerns as well as proposed modifications of the intervention prior to their implementation. Action plans also must be fluid and flexible to accommodate changes in the problem as well as changes in the community. They are revised as circumstances change, and the component action steps will change as well. The plan should be distributed to the entire coalition membership and revisited on a regular basis. The plan also must be unambiguous so that it is well understood by the coalition and easily communicated by each one of them. The plan and its action steps should be the logical outcome of and reflect the overarching goal, vision, mission, objectives, and strategies.

Suggested Activity

Using information from the community culture inquiry, identify three system level action steps to address the identified problem/issue.

Community Health Issue

Long term goal

Short term outcomes

Potential actions/intervention(s)

Action Step	Person(s) Responsible	Date to Be Completed	Resources Required	Plan for Barriers and Resistance	Collaborators

IMPLEMENT

Appealing for support is only part of the implementation process. Neglecting to attend to those who are opposed or even those who are neutral jeopardizes the initiative—particularly if the opposition is organizing for counter action. The most effective implementation process identifies not only those who will support the plan, but also those who will resist, their reasons for resisting, and the influence they have in the community. Special discounts and personal shopping services provided by some grocers or pharmacies, for example, may generate complaints from competitors. Both supporters and opponents are embedded in the social and economic structures that make up the local culture. By understanding the cultural underpinnings of objections, it may be possible to construct a trade-off or compromise, or even a win-win that will satisfy everyone. A creative long term care facility, for example, could develop products and services that actually permit individuals to stay in their own homes as long as possible while at the same time cultivating the loyalty of individuals and families so that when they do need full-time skilled-nursing care, it will be in the facility of choice.

The neutral category of community members is equally significant when organizing for action. These are the groups and individuals who have—or believe they have—nothing to gain or lose in the proposed plan and are, therefore, indifferent. This category of community members is particularly important because support derived from the neutral group may be essential for the project's approval. Moreover, irresolute individuals and groups could be just as easily persuaded to join the opposition. By including neutral but powerful individuals and organizations in the coalition, neutrality or even apathy may be transformed into commitment. Once again, allies, opponents, and neutrals do not remain the same, but shift in relation to the problem at hand. Just because the bus-transit system supports a program for disability accommodation doesn't mean it will support a reduction in fares for seniors. The goal is to articulate and balance competing segments of the community to accomplish a healthy community agenda. Such score cards of trade-offs are the stuff of community public health politics.

In any case, it is essential to not be lulled into a false sense of security by the inherent logic and goodness of the proposal. Even though it may make public health sense, it is unlikely a particular behavior or institution would continue to flourish if someone did not stand to gain from it. Therefore, it is best to anticipate that there will be opposition to even the most modest and seemingly rational change, and to prepare for it accordingly. Ironically, deterrents to change often may come from health professional groups that have a vested interest in maintaining existing services. School nurses, for example, have reported encountering opposition from pediatricians to school based health programs that offer free sports physicals.

TRACK

Having a plan for regular evaluation to track implementation of the healthy community agenda is important to assess progress, analyze trends over time, and evaluate program objectives and progress toward the long term goals. In clinical practice, measuring criteria such as body temperature, redness, or swelling tells us whether the treatment for infection has been effective. This is true of community health practice as well. Once the action plan has been identified and endorsed, the coalition must decide on measureable targets, including how progress will be measured, a timeline for measurement, and the procedures that will be employed. Compared with clinical practice, however, the length of time ordinarily required to see results of community interventions is much longer.

Healthy People 2020 identifies questions that should be answered in a plan for regular evaluations to track implementation of the action plan:

- Did we follow the plan?

- What did we change?

- Did we reach our goal?

Process evaluation occurs throughout implementation of the healthy community agenda and provides the opportunity to change the direction of initiatives and interventions if they are not going as expected, there are untoward effects, resources change, expectations are not being met, or other strategies are deemed more appropriate to the community. Outcome evaluation, on the other hand, is centered on achievement of the healthy community agenda goals and outcomes. Although evaluation is often portrayed as occurring after the plan is in place and underway, in actuality, process- and outcome-evaluation criteria are identified and incorporated into the plan early and throughout the process.

Suggested Activity

Based on your community culture and health assessments, identify short term outcomes and long term goals to meet the healthy community agenda.

Action Plan Activities	Short Term Outcomes to Meet Activity Objectives	Short Term Outcome Measures	Dates to Be Completed	Long Term Goal	Long Term Goal Measures	Date to Be Completed

Finally, the objectives and strategies of a healthy community agenda should offer the most cost-effective solution to the problem. Cost-effectiveness is not synonymous with least expensive. Rather, it gives consideration to the relationship between cost and quality. For one intervention to be considered more cost-effective than another, it must provide equal outcomes at a lower cost or better outcomes at the same cost. Cost must be measured not only in terms of dollars and cents, but in the hidden expenditures of productivity, time, and psychological tolls that are more difficult to monetize. While the initial expense for a project may be high, its maintenance may require little investment. On the other hand, a plan with lower startup costs could ultimately prove to be a more expensive alternative in the long run. It could be argued, for example, that a preliminary analysis of the community's culture is too time-consuming. Yet a plan that is consistent with the cultural expectations and conditions of the community can avoid time-consuming and expensive mistakes. There also are costs incurred if such a program is *not* implemented.

Northville and Southfield: Examples of Culturally Informed Community Action

A comparison of two communities, fictitiously called Northville and Southfield, located in the same rural county, reveals the way in which the position and role of the target groups in their communities influence the configuration of an action plan that is part of a healthy community agenda including the coalition, the assessment data, the short and long range activities, the implementation strategies, and the metric to be achieved.

Nurses from the county decided to seek fiscal support from its 20 towns to extend health promotion, preventive, and health maintenance services to the growing population of elders. Each of the towns already provided a range of well-child services, administered by public health nurses. The services included post-natal visits to high-risk families, parenting classes, child-development programs, and nutrition programs, as well as immunizations, physical exams, and auditory and vision screenings. These programs were administered in collaboration with the schools and supported with funds derived partly from the state and partly from the collection of town tax revenues. The proposed plan would expand public health services to elders and add health education, recreational programs, and community safety to the annual flu-prevention programs.

Southfield is a rural farming community with a population of about 2,100 people, of which almost 300 are over the age of 65. Northville, a neighboring community, has a population of about 2,600, of which approximately 250 are over the age of 65. In spite of the demographic similarities between the towns and their geographic proximity, the proposal for a commitment to elder services was accepted readily by elected officials in Southfield but rejected in Northville.

An examination of the role and status of the elder population (the primary target) in each community provides some clues to explain the difference in commitment to the program by each community. Southfield is a farming community in which elders continue to work in some capacity on family-operated farms, assuming, for example, household and child-care responsibilities. Although they may be less active than their children and/or grand-children in farm operations, they typically are the owners of the farms that succeeding generations will inherit. For the most part, the social life of Southfield is intergenerational and organized around the network of extended families that comprise the population of the town. In addition to their central economic roles as owners of the farms, elders continue to take an active role as leaders in town government, church functions, and community social activities, such as the annual fair or the annual pancake breakfast sponsored by the volunteer firefighters.

Northville resembles Southfield in physical appearance and would be classified as rural by most standards. Only a small segment of the Northville population still engages in farming, however. Most of the land is rented to farmers in surrounding communities, such as Southfield. Much of the population is employed at the large, prestigious Valley Preparatory School tucked into the hills surrounding the center of town. Because residence in Northville entitles local children to tuition benefits as day students at Valley School, many young families have moved to Northville but commute daily to work in the county seat, located 15 miles away. A few of the elders in this community are senior members of farm families, as in Southfield, but most are retired members of the faculty and staff from the preparatory school. Unlike the elders in Southfield, most Northville elders live far from their sons and daughters, who typically are professionals living in other parts of the country. The social and recreational activities in Northville are much more age-segregated, in which the various generations mix only infrequently. Although both the retired and the younger men engage in golf as a pastime, the seniors use a local nine-hole course while the younger men travel to a more-sophisticated golf club in the county seat that puts them in contact with their daily business associates.

In comparison with the Southfield elders, those in Northville were not well integrated with the other generations. They played almost no role in town government, which generally was controlled by the younger generation, and had little economic authority in the community. Seniors simply were not a high priority in Northville. There was even occasional resentment expressed regarding senior residents who continued to occupy large homes in a community where spacious houses were much in demand by young families with children. Essentially, Northville elders had less authority and fewer advocates than their Southfield counterparts.

This example demonstrates that it is not just the size and nature of the target group but its role and status in relation to the rest of the community—particularly the power structure. In Southfield, where elders were comparatively powerful, town officials readily accepted and implemented the proposal. In Northville, on the other hand, where there was no clearly visible base of support for the retired members of the community, the first step was to identify those groups and individuals who would constitute a coalition.

An analysis of the position of elder community members in relation to the cultural context of Northville revealed various points at which elders did, in fact, intersect with other age groups. First, while they were not great in number, there were a few extended farm families in which grandparents and great-grandparents played a significant role. Second, the Congregational Church, in which some retired faculty members from Valley School served as Sunday-school teachers, was one of the few community domains in which intergenerational activities and relationships had developed and flourished—particularly among the women. Third, as leader of a major "industry" in Northville, the headmaster of Valley School was considered to be one of the more influential members of the community.

From this analysis, a Northville coalition was formed that included the following people:

- The minister of the Congregational Church
- A well-liked mother whose child attended Sunday school at the church and whose husband happened to be an elected town official
- A respected farmer whose extended family, including his father, lived on the family farm
- An articulate retired Valley School faculty member

Together, they visited the headmaster of Valley School to ask for his support in convincing town-council members to provide revenue for the project. His own political leverage stemmed from the school's role as a major employer in the community and from its generous tuition benefits to town children. In the meantime, the wife of the town official convinced her husband to reverse his original opinion on the project, and the much-beloved and highly influential minister asked his parishioners for their endorsement. By developing a strategy grounded in knowledge of community culture, this strategically selected coalition was able to overcome the original opposition and secure the resources needed to acquire the commitment of town revenues for promoting the health of seniors.

FORMULATING A CULTURALLY EFFECTIVE COMMUNITY CASE STATEMENT

In clinical practice, nurses carefully present their recommendations in a manner that will ensure their patients' understanding of the importance of the treatment and their engagement in it. This requires individualizing the plan so it is consistent with the lifestyle and values of the specific patient and his or her family. Similarly, in preparing to convince a community of the advisability of system level action, we must construct a message that is framed within the cultural experience of the community, thus converting a professionally identified problem or issue to a culturally defined demand. The goal is to create awareness in the community to generate public action. Whether we are trying to improve the living conditions of seasonal workers, control solid waste, or limit smoking in public places, without this public consciousness-raising, community residents may have little interest in the program, either as a primary or secondary target. Global warming, school violence, child obesity, HIV/AIDS, disaster preparedness, and violence against women have captured the attention of the public, creating a public demand for their resolution. Not surprisingly, simply creating a healthy future for the community may not be a sufficiently powerful motivator for public action without specific action objectives (better schools for children, improved public transportation, beautification of the downtown, safer neighborhoods) that will resonate with the community members. The argument that automobile emissions are contributing to the gradual reduction of the ozone layer, for example, simply may not be as compelling to individuals and families as the prospect of losing a job within the next six months because of new regulations governing the disposal of industrial wastes.

Given the diversity of the community and the presence of proponents, opponents, and neutrals in almost all capacity building agendas, the community appeal is likely to contain more than one message. Some sectors of the community, for example, will respond very well to the argument that regulating the disposal of industrial wastes will result in a healthier environment for future generations. Others will see such an effort as endangering their economic livelihood by regulating the industries in which they work. Still others will be indifferent. In a diverse community, the message and the action plan must be segmented to address the various goals and values present in the community we are attempting to persuade.

In addition to a culturally appropriate and segmented message, the case statement must include all of the critical information related to the issue so that everyone who is promoting the community action is well-prepared to defend it. In explaining their support of controversial legislation, politicians, for example, must have compelling justification regarding both the costs as well as the benefits to their constituents both now and in the future. The community case statement consists of the following:

■ The overarching goal, which the action plan supports

■ A statement of the problem (what is the issue/concern?)

■ The magnitude of the problem (the number and characteristics of the individuals and families in the community who are or will be affected—both directly and indirectly)

■ The cost of the issue/problem to the community (what is the impact, and at what cost?)

■ The proposed action

■ The projected outcomes

■ The cost to the community of *not* taking this action

The community case statement should be generated by the coalition and then designed and used to inform all relevant segments of the community so that everyone involved will be working toward the same goal with the same information, even if it might be for different reasons.

The goal of the case statement is to convince and persuade; therefore, all information must be accurate, reliable, and understandable to all segments of the community. Statistics and statements of fact must be current and compiled from credible sources, checked, and rechecked. Even the most minor math error detracts from the credibility of the document and its authors. Because those who are not in favor of the proposed change will examine the statement carefully in an attempt to discredit the message, the facts must be accurate and the argument logical to defend the statement and counter opposition.

Finding a proper balance of statistical data and qualitative description will depend on the characteristics of the audience. Because we live in a society that has confidence in science and numbers, statistical evidence is useful but should be selected carefully to make a point. Less scientific, but sometimes more convincing, are human-interest data that have an emotional appeal. A description of one or two actual cases (having first gained permission from those involved to share this information) often will be more persuasive than the statistics derived from a study of hundreds of families. Thus, while it is necessary to have on hand an objective, rational argument about why a specific plan would improve the health of the community, an emotional appeal can be extraordinarily effective, even with the most conservative audience. For example, although figures stating that millions of tax dollars spent on drug abuse each year constitute important evidence, they are somehow less real than the case of a family that lost its home and savings because of drug abuse by one of its members. The plight of real people is something with which most everyone can identify.

In conclusion, the overarching goal of public health practice is a healthy community—that is, a physical, economic, and social infrastructure with the capacity to mobilize material and social resources and protect the growth and sustainability of community life. Although much of public health practice is focused on the action plan, the strategy for achieving our overarching goal is not just implementing a collection of unrelated community initiatives but rather implementing an integrated, comprehensive healthy community agenda. Through civic action, we work with community residents to enhance the community's capacity to protect and promote the health of citizens now and in the future.

REFERENCES

Alinsky, S. (1971). *Rules for Radicals*. New York, NY: Vintage Books, Random House.

American Lung Association. (2010). State of the air 2010: Key findings. *American Lung Association*. Retrieved February 17, 2011, from http://stateoftheair.org/

American Nurses Association. (2007). *Public Health Nursing: Scope and Standards of Practice*. Silver Spring, MD: Author.

Andrews, M., & Boyle, J. (2008). *Transcultural concepts in nursing care*. Philadelphia, PA: Lippincott Williams & Wilkins.

Arensberg, C. (1961). The community as object and sample. *American Anthropologist*; 63.2 (1961): 241–264.

Arensberg, C., & Kimball, S. (1965). *Culture and community*. New York: Harcourt, Brace, and World.

Armelagos, G. J., Brown, P. J., & Turner, B. (2005). Evolutionary, historical and political Economic Perspectives on Health and Disease. *Social Science and Medicine* 61: 755–65.

Azevedo-Garcia, D., Lochner, K. A., Osypuk, T. L., & Subramanian, S. V. (2003). Future directions in residential segregation and health research: A multilevel approach. *American Journal of Public Health* 93.2: 215–220.

Bender, A., Clune, L., & Guruge, S. (2009). Considering place in community health nursing. *Canadian Journal of Nursing Research*, 41(1): 128–43.

Benkert, R., Tanner, C., Guthrie, B., Oakley, D., & Pohl, J. M. (2005). Cultural competence of nurse practitioner students: A consortium's experience. *Journal of Nursing Education* 44.5: 225–233.

Berkman, L. F., & Syme, L. S. (1979). Social networks, host resistance, and mortality: A nine-year follow-up study of Alameda County residents. *American Journal of Epidemiology* 109.2: 186–204.

Bernard, H. R. (2011). Research methods in anthropology: Qualitative andqQuantitativeaApproaches. 5th ed. Lanham, MD: AltaMira Press.

Betancourt, J. R., Green, A. R., Carrillo, J. E., & Ananeh-Firempong, O., 2nd. (2003). Defining cultural competence: A practical framework for addressing racial/ethnic disparities in health and health care. *Public Health Reports* 118.4 (2003): 293–302.

Bibeau, G. (1997). At work in the fields of public health: The abuse of rationality. *Anthropology Quarterly* 11.2: 246–255.

Bloom, B., Cohen, R., & Freeman, G. (2008). Summary health statistics for U.S. children: National health interview survey, 2008. National Center for Health Statistics, *Vital Health Statistics*. Series 10, No. 244: 1–81.

Buhler-Wilkerson, K. (1993). Bringing care to the people: Lillian Wald's legacy to public health nursing. *American Journal of Public Health;* 83(12): 1778–1786.

Burgard, S. A., Brand, J. E., & House, J. S. (2007). Toward a better estimation of the effect of job loss on health. *Journal of Health and Social Behavior* 48: 369–84.

Butterfield, P. (1990). Thinking upstream: Nurturing a conceptual understanding of the societal context of health behavior. *Advances in Nursing Science* 12.2 1–8.

Butterfield, P. (2002). Upstream reflections on environmental health. *Advances in Nursing Science* 21.1: 32–49.

Campinha-Bacote, J. & Munoz, C. (2001). A guiding framework for delivering culturally competent services in case management. *The Case Manager* 12.2: 48–52.

Carlson, E., & Chamberlain, R. (2004). The black-white perception gap and health disparities research. *Public Health Nursing* 21.4 (2004): 372–379.

Carolan, M., Andrews, G. J., & Hodnett, E. (2006). Writing place: A comparison of nursing research and health geography. Nursing Inquiry 13(3): 203–19.

Centers for Disease Control and Prevention, Core Public Health Functions Steering Committee. (2010). National public health performance standards program: Orientation to the essential public health services. Author. Retrieved March 31, 2011, from http://www.cdc.gov/nphpsp/essentialServices.html

Centers for Disease Control and Prevention, National Center for Injury Prevention and Control. (2011). Web-based injury statistics query and reporting system (WISQARS). Author. Retrieved March 30, 2011, from http://www.cdc.gov/injury/wisqars

Centers for Disease Control and Prevention. (2011). Chronic disease prevention and health promotion. Author. Retrieved January 27, 2011, from http://www.cdc.gov/chronicdisease/index.htmc

Chafey, K. (1996). "Caring" is not enough: Ethical paradigms for community-based care. *Nursing and Health Care Perspectives on Community* 17.1: 10–15.

Clancy, K. J., Berger, P. D., & Magliozzi, T. L. (2003). The ecological fallacy: Some fundamental research misconceptions corrected. *Journal of Advertising Research* 43: 370–380.

Clark, M. (2007). *Community health nursing: Advocacy for population health* (5th edition) . Upper Saddle River, New Jersey: Prentice Hall.

Corin, E. (1994). The social and cultural matrix of health and disease. In *Why are some people healthy and others not? The determinants of health of populations* (Robert G. Evans, Morris L. Barer, and Theodore R. Marmor, eds.). New York, NY: A. de Gruyter.

Cummins, S., Curtis, S., Diez-Roux, A. V., & Macintyre, M. (2007). Understanding and representing "place" in health research: A relational approach. *Social Science & Medicine*, 65(9): 1825–1838.

Cummins, S., Stafford, M., Macintyre, S., Marmot, M., & Ellaway, A. (2005). Neighborhood environment and its association with self rated health: Evidence from Scotland and England. *Journal of Epidemiology and Community Health;* 59(3): 207–213.

Cuzick, J. (2003). Epidemiology of breast cancer—selected highlights. *Breast* 12.6: 405–411.

Davis, R. (2000). Holographic community: Reconceptualizing the meaning of community in an era of health care reform. *Nursing Outlook* 48.6: 295–301.

Dreher, M. (1982a).The conflict of conservatism in public health nursing education. *Nursing Outlook* 30.9: 504–509.

Dreher, M. (1982b). *Working Men and Ganja.* Philadelphia, PA: ISHI Publications.

Dreher, M. (1984). District nursing: The cost benefits of a community-based practice. *American Journal of Public Health.* 74.10: 1107–1111.

Dreher, M. (1996). Nursing: A cultural phenomenon. *Reflections on Nursing Leadership* 1.4: 4.

Dreher, M., & Hudgins, R. (2010). Maternal conjugal multiplicity and child development in rural Jamaica. *Family Relations* 59.5: 495–505.

Dreher, M., & MacNaughton, N. (2002). Cultural competence in nursing: fallacy or foundation? *Nursing Outlook* 50.5: 181–186.

Dressler, W. W. (1982). Hypertension and culture change: Acculturation and disease in the West Indies. South Salem, NY: Redgrave.

Dressler, W. W. (2004). Culture and the risk of disease. *British Medical Bulletin* 69.1: 21–31.

Dressler, William W. (1985) The social and cultural context of coping: action, gender, and symptoms in a Southern black community. *Social Science and Medicine* 21: 499-506.

Drevdahl, D. (1995). Coming to voice: The power of emancipatory community interventions. *Advances in Nursing Science* 18.2 : 13–24.

Drevdahl, D. (1999). Meanings of community in a community health center. *Public Health Nursing* 16(6): 375-440.

Drevdahl, D. J. (2002). Home and border: The contradictions of community. *Advances in Nursing Science* 24.3: 8–20.

Drevdahl, D., Philips, D., & Taylor, J. (2006). Uncontested categories: The use of race and ethnicity variables in nursing research. *Nursing Inquiry* 13.1: 53–63.

Dubos, R. (1965). *Man adapting.* New Haven, CT: Yale University Press.

DuRant, R. H., Cadenhead, C., Pendergrast, R. A., Slavens, G., & Linder, C. W. (1994). Factors associated with the use of violence among urban black adolescents. *American Journal of Public Health* 84.4: 612–617.

Eberhardt, M., & Pamuk, E. (2004). The importance of place of residence: Examining health in rural and non-rural areas. *American Journal of Public Health* 94.10: 1682–1686.

Edelson, M. (2008). Culturally attuned messages delivered by peers may be the best way to stop HIV from surging among at-risk, hidden populations. *Johns Hopkins Public Health Magazine.* Retrieved March 31, 2011, from http://magazine.Jhsph.edu/2008/Spring/culture/living

Everly, G. S., Jr., & Flynn, B. W. (2006). Principles and practical procedures for acute psychological first aid training for personnel without mental health experience. *International Journal of Emergency Mental Health* 8(2): 93–100.

Fahrenwald, N., Boysen, R., Fischer, C., & Maurer, R. (2001). Developing cultural competence in the baccalaureate nursing student: A population-based project with the Hutterites. *Journal of Transcultural Nursing* 12.1: 48–55.

Fahrenwald, N., Taylor, J., Kneipp, S., & Canales, M. (2007). Academic freedom and academic duty to teach social justice: A perspective and pedagogy for public health nursing faculty. *Public Health Nursing* 24.2: 190–197.

Feld, M.(2008). *Lillian Wald: A biography.* Chapel Hill, NC: University of North Carolina Press.

Freeman, R. (1963). *Public health nursing practice*. 3rd ed. Philadelphia, PA: Saunders.

Friedman, T. (2008). *Hot, flat and crowded*. New York, NY: Farrar, Straus and Giroux.

Gehlbach, S. (2005). American plagues: Lessons from our battles with disease. New York, NY: McGraw-Hill Professional.

Grunberg, L., Moore, S., Sikora, P., & Greenberg, E. (2008). The changing workplace and its effects: Employee attitudinal and behavioral responses over time at a large american company. *Journal of Applied Behavioral Science* 44.2: 215–236.

Hammett, T. M., Harmon, M. P., & Rhodes, W. (2002). The burden of infectious disease among inmates of and releases from U.S. correctional facilities, 1997. *American Journal of Public Health* 92.11: 1789–1794.

Hebel, J. R., & McCarter, R. J. (2006). *A study guide to epidemiology and biostatistics*. 6th ed. Sudbury, MA: Jones and Bartlett Learning.

Helman, C. (2007). *Culture, health, and illness*. London: Hodder Arnold.

Henry Street Settlement. (n.d.). Lillian Wald. *Henry Street Settlement*. Retrieved on March 31, 2011, from http://www.henrystreet.org/about/history/lillian-wald.html

Heymann, J., Hertzman, C., Barer, M., & Evans, R. (2006). *Healthier societies: From analysis to action*. Oxford: Oxford University Press.

Hopkins, N., & Mehanna, S. R. (2000). Social action against everyday pollution in Egypt. *Human Organization* 59.2: 245–254.

Hopkins, N., & Mehanna, S. R. (2003). Living with pollution in Egypt. *The Environmentalist* 23.1: 17–28.

Institute of Medicine. (2008*). Retooling for an aging America: Building the health care workforce*. Washington, D.C.: National Academies Press.

Institute of Medicine. (2010*).The future of nursing: Leading change, advancing health*. Washington, D.C.: National Academies Press.

Kaiser Family Foundation. (2006). Race, ethnicity and health care fact sheet: Young African American men in the United States. *Kaiser Family Foundation*. Retrieved January 21, 2011, by http://www.kff.org/minorityhealth/upload/7541.pdf

Keene, D., Padilla, M., & Geronimus, A. (2010). Leaving Chicago for Iowa's fields of opportunity: Community dispossession, rootlessness, and the quest for somewhere to be OK. *Human Organization* 69.3: 275–284.

Kerker, B., Bainbridge, J., Kennedy, J., Bennani, Y., Agerton, T., Marder, D. et al. (2011). A population-based assessment of the health of homeless families in New York City, 2001-2003. *American Journal of Public Health*, 101(3): 545–553.

Koplan, J. P., Bond, T. C., Merson, M. H., Reddy, K. S., Rodriguez, M. H., Sewankam-bo, N. K. et al. (2008). Towards a common definition of global health. Lancet 6.373: 1993–5.

Krause, N. (2002). Church-based social support and health in old age. *The Journals of Gerontology* Series B. Social Sciences 57.6: S332–347.

Kreuter, M., & McClure, S. (2004). The role of culture in health communication. *Annual Review of Public Health* 25: 439–455.

Kung, H. C., Hoyert, D. L., Xu J. Q., & Murphy, S. L. (2008). Deaths: Final data for 2005. *National Vital Statistics Reports* 56.10. Available from http://www.cdc.gov/nchs/data/nvsr/nvsr56/nvsr56_10.pdf

Leininger, M. (1989). Leininger's theory of nursing: Cultural care diversity and universality. *Nursing Science Quarterly* 1.4: 152–160.

Leininger, M. (1997). Transcultural nursing research to transform nursing education and practice. *Image: Journal of Nursing Scholarship* 29: 341–347.

Levine, A. (1982). *Love Canal: Science, politics, and people.* Lexington, MA: Lexington Books.

Marmot, M. (2005). The social environment and health. *Journal of the Royal College of Physicians*, 5(3): 244–248.

Marmot, M. (2009). Social determinants of health inequalities. *Lancet*, 365(9464): 1099–1104.

McElroy, A., & Townsend, P. (2004). *Medical anthropology in ecological perspective.* New York, NY: Westview Press.

McKay, M. L., & Hewlett, P. O. (2009). Grassroots coalition building: Lessons from the field. *Journal of Professional Nursing*, 25.6: 352–357.

McMichael, A. J. (2001). Frontiers, environments, and Disease: Past patterns, uncertain futures. Cambridge: Cambridge University Press.

Milio, N. (1970). *9226 Kercheval Street: The storefront that did not burn.* Ann Arbor, MI: University of Michigan Press.

Milio, N. (1975). *The care of health in communities.* New York, NY: MacMillan.

Minkler, M. (2005). *Community organizing and community building for health.* Newark, NJ: Rutgers University Press.

National Center for Health Statistics. (2011). Health, United States. Hyattsville, MD.

National Heart, Lung, and Blood Institute and Boston University. (2011). Framingham Heart Study. Retrieved on March 31, 2011, from http://www.framinghamheartstudy.org/index.html

National Research Council of the National Academies. (2003). Elder mistreatment: Abuse, neglect, and exploitation in an aging america: Panel to review risk and prevalence of elder abuse and neglect. Bonnie, R.J. & Wallace, R.B. Washington D.C.: National Academies Press.

Newton, L., & Smith, D. (2004). *Wake-up calls: Classic cases in business ethics*. Mason, OH: Thomson/South-Western.

Office of National Drug Control Policy. (2006). Drug-related crime March 2000. *ONDCP Drug Policy Information Clearinghouse Fact Sheet*. Retrieved February 17, 2011, from http://www.whitehousedrugpolicy.gov/publications/factsht/crime/index. html

Ogden, C., & Carroll, M. (2010). NCHS health e-stat: Prevalence of obesity among children and adolescents: United States, Trends 1963–1965 through 2007–2008. *Centers for Disease Control and Prevention*. Retrieved April 2, 2011, from http://www.cdc.gov/nchs/data/hestat/obesity_child_07_08/obesity_child_07_08.htm.

Omeri, A., & Malcolm, P. (2004). Cultural diversity: A challenge for community nurses. *Contemporary Nurse* 17.3 (2004): 183–191.

Paul, B., ed. (1955). Health, culture, community: Case studies of public reactions to health programs. New York, NY: Russell Sage Foundation.

Peterson, J., Atwood, J., & Yates, B. (2002). Key elements for church-based health promotion programs: Outcome-based literature review. *Public Health Nursing* 19.6: 410–411.

Phillips, D., & Drevdahl, D. (2003). Race and the difficulties of language. *Advances in Nursing Science* 26.1: 17–29.

Public Health Foundation. (2010). Core competencies for public health. *Public Health Foundation*. Retrieved January 27, 2011, from http://www.phf.org/resourcestools/Pages/Core_Public_Health_Competencies.aspx

Quad Council of Public Health Nursing Organizations. (2004). Public health nursing competencies. *Public Health Nursing* 21.5: 443–452.

Racher, F., & Annis, R. (2007). Respecting culture and honoring diversity in community practice. *Research and Theory in Nursing Practice* 2.14: 255–70.

Reagan, P. B., & Salsberry, P. J. (2005). Race and ethnic differences in determinants of preterm birth in the USA: Broadening the social context. *Social Science and Medicine* 60: 2217–2228.

Roberts, E. (1997). Neighborhood social environments and the distribution of low birth weight in Chicago. *American Journal of Public Health* 87.4: 597–603.

Rodwin, V., & Neuberg, L. (2005). Infant mortality and income in 4 world cities: New York, London, Paris and Tokyo. *American Journal of Public Health* 95.1: 86–90.

Rosen, G. (1954). The community and the health officer: A working team. *American Journal of Public Health* 44.1: 14–17.

Rothman, J. (2008). Strategies of community intervention. J. Rothman (Ed.) Peosta, Iowa: Eddie Bowers Pub.

Sikora, P., Moore, S., Greenberg, E., & Grunberg, L. (2008). Downsizing and alcohol use: A cross-lagged longitudinal examination of the Sspillover hypothesis. *Work & Stress* 22.1: 51–68.

Simmons, A, Reynolds, R. & Swinburn, B. (2011). Defining community-capacity building: Is it possible? *Preventive Medicine* 52: 193-199.

Stafford, M. & Marmot, M. (2003). Neighbourhood deprivation and health: Does it affect us all equally? *International Journal of Epidemiology*, (32): 357–366.

Steckler, A. B., & Herzog, W. T. (1979). How to keep your mandated citizen board out of your hair and off your back: A guide for executive directors. *American Journal of Community Health* 69.8: 809–812.

Strawbridge, W., Cohen, R., Shema, S., & Kaplan, G. (1997). Frequent attendance at religious services and mortality over 28 years. *American Journal of Public Health* 87.6: 957–961.

Szwarcwald, C. L., Correa da Mota, J., Damacena, G. M., & Pereira, T. G. S. (2011). Health inequalities in Rio de Janeiro, Brazil: Lower healthy life expectancy in socioeconomically disadvantaged areas. *American Journal of Public Health;* 101(3): 517–523.

Tarlier, D., Browne, A. J., & Johnson, J. (2007). The influence of geographical and social distance on nursing practice and continuity of care in a remote First Nations community. *Canadian Journal of Nursing Research*, 39(3): 126–48.

Tripp-Reimer, T. (1999). Cultural interventions for ethnic groups of color in *Handbook of Clinical Nursing Research*, Hinshaw, A.S., Feetham, S. & Shaver, J. eds. Thousand Oaks, CA: Sage.

Tripp-Reimer, T., Choi, E., Skemp-Kelley, L., & Enslein, J. (2001). Cultural barriers to care: Inverting the problem. *Diabetes Spectrum* 14.1: 13–22.

U.S. Census Bureau. (2008a). *2008 American Community Survey*. Retrieved November 7, 2010, from http://factfinder.census.gov

U.S. Census Bureau. (2008b). Population estimates: National characteristics: National sex, age, race, and Hispanic origin. *U.S. Census Bureau*. Retrieved March 22, 2011, from http://www.census.gov/popest/national/asrh/NC-EST2008-asrh.html

United Nations. (2010). Water Scarcity. *International Decade for Action: Water for Life, 2005–2015*. Retrieved March 25, 2011, from http://www.un.org/waterforlifedecade/scarcity.html

United States Department of Health and Human Services. (2011). *Healthy People 2020*. HealthyPeople.gov. Retrieved March 23, 2011, from http://www.healthypeople.gov

United States Department of Health and Human Services. Office of Minority Health. (2010). *The National Plan for Action Draft*. National Partnership for Action to End Health Disparities. Retrieved April 5, 2011, from http://www.minorityhealth.hhs.gov/npa/templates/browse.aspx?&lvl=2&lvlid=34

United States Department of Health and Human Services.(2001). Cultural competence works. Using cultural competence to improve the quality of health care for diverse populations and add value to managed care arrangements. Merrifield, VA.

United States Department of Health and Human Services.(2001). *Healthy People 2010*. McLean, VA: International Medical Publishing, Inc.

Wald, L. (1934). *Windows on Henry Street*. Boston, MA: Little Brown and Company.

Webb, B., Simpson, S., & Hairston, L. (2011). From politics to parity: Using a health disparities index to guide legislative efforts for health equity. *American Journal of Public Health* 101.3: 554–559.

Wellin, E. (1955). Water boiling in a Peruvian town. *Health, culture, and community*. New York, NY: Russell Sage Foundation.

Whitaker, E. D. (2003). The idea of health: History, medical pluralism, and the management of the body in Emilia-Romagna, Italy. *Medical Anthropology Quarterly* 17.3): 348–375.

White, K. L. (1973). Life and death and medicine. *Scientific American* 229.3: 23–33.

Williamson, M., & Harrison, L. (2010). Providing culturally appropriate care: A literature review. *International Journal of Nursing Studies*, 47.6: 761–769.

Wolf, E. (1994). Perilous ideas: Race, culture, people. *Current Anthropology* 35.1: 1–12.

Woodruff, T. J., Zota, A.R., & Schwartz, J. M. (2011). Environmental chemicals in pregnant women in the U.S. *Environmental Health Perspectives*, 119(6):878-85.

World Health Organization. (2007). Global age-friendly cities: A guide. World Health Organization. Retrieved January 25, 2011, from http://www.who.int/ageing/publications/Global_age_friendly_cities_Guide_English.pdf

World Health Organization. (2011). Ageing. World Health Organization. Retrieved March 31, 2011, from http://www.who.int/topics/ageing/en

Worthman, C. M., & Kohrt, B. (2005). Receding horizons of health: Biocultural approaches to public health paradoxes. *Social Science and Medicine* 61: 861–878.

Young Laing, B. (2009) A critique of Rothman's and other standard community organizing models: Toward developing a culturally proficient community organizing framework. *Community Development Society*, (40): 17-20.

INDEX

A

adolescent health, 160
advisory board, 206–207
agencies
    health departments, 173–174
    health planning, 174–175
    personal health care, 174
agenda creation, 193
    action plan, 218–224
    community engagement,
      196–198
    mission, 194–196
    objectives, 198–202
    overarching goals, 194
    stakeholders, 196–198
    strategies, 202–205
    value statements, 195–196
    values, 194–196
    vision, 194–196
alternative health systems,
    178–179
anthropology, 48–49
    community development
      and, 76
    community health nursing,
      14–15
    social services and, 76
assertiveness of nurses, 17
assessment of community,
    26–27, 36
asthma, 30

B

behavioral health, 156
beliefs and values, 177–178
biological composition of
    population, 96–98
bio-statistics, 37–38
    calculating rates, 38–40
    crude rates, 39–40
    morbidity rates, 41–42
    mortality rates, 40–41
    odds ratios, 44
birth, 37–38
bisexual persons. *See* LBGT
    health
book's premises, 18

C

caring, public health and,
    16–17
case statement, 237–240
case-control studies, 43–45
categorical programs, 21
causal relationships, 47
CDC (Centers for Disease
    Control and Prevention), 61
child health, 157–159
chronic disability, 154–155
chronic diseases, 153–154

civic action. *See* community action
clients, 22–24
climate factors of community, 80–81
coalitions, 224–225
cohort studies, 45–47
communication in community, 85–86
community
    capacity, 24–25
    as client, 19
    coordination, 30–31
    cyclical crises, 92–93
    data gathering, 50–51
        direct observation, 52–55
        documentation, 57–60
        member information, 55–56
    definition, 10
    economic cycles, 90
    engagement in agenda planning, 196–198
    ethnic structure, 28
    evaluation, 31
    health analysis, 68–73
    history, 87–88
    influential residents, 206
    nurse-community relationship, 31–33
    nurses as residents, 217
    physical environment, 7–8
        spatial dimensions, 77–87
    population, 7, 8–9, 93
        age, 96–98
        biological composition, 96–98
        density, 94
        distribution, 94
        education level, 100–101
        ethnic groups, 98–100

        household characteristics, 102–103, 109
        income, 100–101
        occupation, 100–101
        racial groups, 98–100
        residential characteristics, 102–103
        sex, 96–98
        size, 94
        temporary subpopulations, 94
    practitioners as members, 216–217
    psychological cycles, 91–92
    social organization, 7, 9–10
        government, 107–123
        institutions, 103–106
        law enforcement, 107–123
        politics, 107–123
community action
    capacity building, 210
    change, 210–212
    citizen engagement, 210
    cultural preservation, 210–212
    models, 212–215
        conflict model, 213–214
        consensus model, 213
    nurses' role, 216–217
community advisory board, 206–207
community case statement, 237–240
community constituencies, building, 205–208
community health, 10–12
    nursing
        anthropology, 14–15
        definition, 20
        epidemiology, 12–14
        origins, 20

orientation, xii
shared responsibility, 197
community health assessment, 126
accidents, 143–144
community buildings, 145–146
crime, 142–143
disease vectors, 139–140
energy management, 147
environmental health, 126–128
food contamination, 132
outdoor air quality, 128–130
water quality, 130–131
global health, 147–149
hazardous waste management, 132
chemical waste, 136–138
sewage, 134
solid waste, 133
homes and communities, 144–145
noise pollution, 138
preparedness, 140–141
toxic substances, 132
chemical waste, 136–138
pesticides, 136–138
radioactive waste, 135–136
community nursing
political conservatism, 16–18
values, 33–34
community practice
clients, 22–24
community assessment, 26–27, 36
community evaluation, 31
goals, 24–26
intervention, 27–30
strategies, 29
planning, 27–30

Community Practice Notebook, 50–51
confidentiality, 32
conflict model for community action,
213–214
consensus model for community action,
213
constituencies, building, 205–208
contemporary public health, 10–11
coordinating services, 30–31
core public health leadership competencies,
xi
crime, 142–143
crude rates of bio-statistics, 39–40
cultural capital, 6
schools as, 25
cultural competence, xiii
description, 3–5
ethnic communities and, 4
H1N1 flu epidemic, 6
in public health, 5–6
cultural phenomenon of nursing, 3
cultural preservation in community action,
210–212
cultural realities, xiv
culturally informed community health
analysis, 68–73
culture
of community, 76
concept, 2–3
as ethnicity, 4
fluidity of, 1
as group characteristic, 4
nursing *versus* medicine, 2
public health nurses, 2

culture based planning, 188–192
cyclical crises of community, 92–93
cyclical movement of population, 89

D

data
    CDC (Centers for Disease Control and
       Prevention), 61
    epidemiological studies, 62–63
    health surveys, 62–63
    Internet sources, 63–67
    local sources, 62
    state health departments, 61–62
    U.S. Census, 60
demand, managing, 185
disability, 154–155
disease vectors, 139–140
district nursing, 20
Dubos, Rene, 11

E

early childhood health, 159–160
economic cycles of community, 90
economic institutions, 105–106
education of community, 112–113
energy management, 147
environment, health and, 127
environmental health, 126–128, 149–150
    food contamination, 132

outdoor air quality, 128–130
    water quality, 130–131
environmental resources, 66–67
epidemiological studies, 62–63
    case-control studies, 43–45
    cohort studies, 45–47
epidemiology
    of community health nursing, 12–14
    risk factors and, 37
ethnic communities, cultural competence
    and, 4
ethnic groups, 98–100
ethnic structure, 28
ethnography, 48–49
    health and illness matrix, 49–50

F

Federal Children's Bureau, 21
financing, 175–176
fluidity of cultures, 1
food safety, contamination, 132
funding, disease-oriented, 21

G

gay persons. *See* LBGT health
geophysical and climate factors, 80–81
global health, 147–149
government of community, 107–123
ground-water quality, 130–131

H

H1N1 flu epidemic, cultural capital, 6
hazardous waste management, 132
   chemical waste, 136–138
   sewage, 134
   solid waste, 133
health
   community health, 10–12
   place and, xii
health care institutions, 168–170
health care organization
   prevention
      primary, 166–167
      secondary, 167
      tertiary, 167–168
   public health services, institutions,
      168–170
health departments, 61–62, 173–174
health surveys, 62–63
health *versus* health care, xi
health planning agencies, 174–175
Healthy People 2020, goals, 18
Henry Street Settlement, 20
high-school completion, 204
history of community, 87–88
horizontal stratification, 118–120
household characteristics of population,
   102–103, 109
housing in community, 83–84

I

immunization, rate increase goal, 23
incidence rates, 41–42
indigenous health services, 178–179
infant birth weight, Chicago, 14
infant health, 157–159
infectious diseases, 152–153
influential residents, 206
information systems, 172
international health resources, 64
Internet, health statistics sources, 63–67
intervention, 27–30
   strategies, 29

L

land use of community, 81–82
law enforcement of community, 107–123
lesbians. *See* LBGT health
LGBT health, 162–163

M

management, demand, 185
MAP-IT framework, 218
   assess, 226–228
   implement, 230–231
   mobilize, 224–225

plan, 228–230
    track, 231–237
maternal health, 157–159
medical anthropology, 14–15
Medicare, 21
mental health, 156
mental maps in community, 86–87
middle childhood health, 159–160
mission in agenda planning, 194–196
mobilization, 224–225
Mobilize, Assess, Plan, Implement, Track.
    See MAP-IT framework
morbidity, 37–38
    rates, 41–42
mortality, 37–38
    rates, 40–41

N

National Health Planning Resources and
    Development Act of 1974, 185
National Organization for Public Health
    Nursing, 21
neighborhoods, 86–87
    subgroups, 120
Nightingale, Florence, community nursing
    and, 20
noise pollution, 138
nurse-community relationship, 31–33
nursing as cultural phenomenon, 3
nursing education, relationships, 17

O

obesity, culture based planning and,
    190–191
occupational safety health, 163–164
odds ratios, 44
organizations, voluntary, 116–118
orientation, xii
outdoor air quality, 128–130

P

Patient Protection and Affordable Care
    Act, xiv
patterns, 27
personal health care agencies, 174
personal health services, 29
physical environment
    community and, 7
    components, 7–8
    spatial dimensions, 77–78
        communication, 85–86
        geophysical and climate factors,
            80–81
        housing, 83–84
        land use, 81–82
        mental maps, 86–87
        population, 78
        regional position, 79–80
        transportation, 84–85
place and health, xii

planning, 27–30
  agenda creation, 193
    action plan, 218–224
    community engagement, 196–198
    mission, 194–196
    objectives, 198–202
    overarching goals, 194
    stakeholders, 196–198
    strategies, 202–205
    values, 194–196
    vision, 194–196
  citizen participation, 197
  culture based, 188–192
  importance of, 183–184
  National Health Planning Resources
    and Development Act of 1974, 185
  population-based, 186–188
  resource-based, 184–186
political conservatism, community nursing
  and, 16–18
politics of community, 107–123
population, 7, 8–9, 93
  age, 96–98
  biological composition, 96–98
  boundaries, 78
  cyclical movement, 89
  density, 94
  distribution, 78, 94
  education level, 100–101
  ethnic groups, 98–100
  geopolitically defined, 23
  household characteristics, 102–103,
    109
  income, 100–101

occupation, 100–101
racial groups, 98–100
residential characteristics, 102–103
sex, 96–98
size, 78, 94
temporary subpopulations, 95
vulnerable populations, 187
population health & behaviors, 164–165
population health assessment, 150–151
  adolescent health, 160
  behavioral health, 156
  child health, 157–159
  chronic disability, 154–155
  chronic diseases, 153–154
  early childhood health, 159–160
  infant health, 157–159
  infectious diseases, 152–153
  LGBT health, 162–163
  maternal health, 157–159
  mental health, 156
  middle childhood health, 159–160
  occupational safety and health,
    163–164
  older adult health, 161–162
  population health & behaviors,
    164–165
population resources, 67
population-based planning, 186–188
populations, health status and, 22
practitioners as community members,
  216–217
preparedness for disaster, 140–141
prevalence rates, 41–42
prevention, 166–168

psychological cycles of community, 91–92
public health
    agencies, 172
        health departments, 173–174
        health planning, 174–175
        personal health care, 174
    caring, 16–17
    cultural competence, 5–6
    data access
        CDC, 61
        epidemiological studies, 62–63
        health surveys, 62–63
        Internet sources, 63–67
        local sources, 62
        state health departments, 61–62
        U.S. Census, 60
    father of contemporary, 11
    financing, 175–176
    information systems, 172
    nurses, culture, 2
    nursing, origins, 20
    values and beliefs, 177–178
    workforce, 171–172
public high-school completion, 204

R

racial groups, 98–100
rates, 27
Rathbone, William, 20
recreation in community, 114–115
regional position of community, 79–80
relationships, nurse-community, 31–33

religion, 110–112
residential characteristics of population,
    102–103
residents
    influential, 206
    nurses in community, 217
resource-based planning, 184–186
resources, Internet, 63–67
role modeling, 32

S

same-sex couples, 110
school nurses, 21
schools as cultural capital, 25
smoking in Rhode Island, 13
social organization of community, 7, 9–10
    education, 112–113
    government, 107–123
    horizontal stratification, 118–120
    institutions, 103–106
    law enforcement, 107–123
    politics, 107–123
    recreation, 114–115
    religion, 110–112
    vertical segmentation, 120–123
    voluntary organizations, 116–118
spatial dimensions of community life,
    77–78
    communication, 85–86
    geophysical and climate factors, 80–81
    housing, 83–84
    land use, 81–82

mental maps, 86–87
population, 78
regional position, 79–80
transportation, 84–85
stakeholders in agenda planning, 196–198
coalitions, 224–225
state health departments, 61–62
state-based resources, 66
subgroups in neighborhoods, 120
surface-water quality, 130–131

T

temporary subpopulations, 95
topic-specific resources, 67
toxic substances, 132
chemical waste, 136–138
pesticides, 136–138
radioactive waste, 135–136
transgendered persons. *See* LBGT health
transportation in community, 84–85
trends, 27

U

urbanization, 126
U.S. Census data, 60
U.S. governmental health resources, 64–66
U.S. national health resources, 64–66

V

value statements in agenda planning, 195–196
values, 33–34
in agenda planning, 194–196
values and beliefs, 177–178
vertical segmentation, 120–123
vision in agenda planning, 194–196
voluntary organizations, 116–118
vulnerable populations, 187

W–Z

Wald, Lillian, 16, 20–21
Windows on Henry Street, 21
water quality, 130–131
Windows on Henry Street (Wald), 21
workforce in public health, 171–172
workplace, health inspections, 21

NOTES

NOTES

NOTES

NOTES

NOTES

NOTES

NOTES

NOTES

NOTES